MRCPCH 1:
Essential Questions in Paediatrics
Second Edition

Dr R M Beattie
BSc MBBS MRCP FRCPCH
Consultant Paediatric Gastroenterologist
Paediatric Medical Unit
Southampton General Hospital
Southampton

Dr M P Champion
BSc MBBS MRCP FRCPCH
Consultant in Paediatric Inherited Metabolic Disease
Evelina Children's Hospital
Guy's and St Thomas' NHS Foundation Trust
London

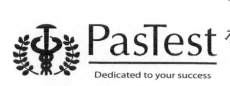

PasTest
Dedicated to your success

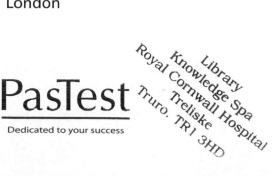

© 2009 PASTEST LTD
Egerton Court
Parkgate Estate
Knutsford
Cheshire, WA16 8DX

Telephone: 01565 752000

A percentage of the material was previously published in *Essential Questions in
Paediatrics for MRCPCH Volume 1* (ISBN 1901198995) and *Volume 2* (ISBN
1904627331)

First published 2009

ISBN: 1905635 532
        978 1905635 535

A catalogue record for this book is available from the British Library.

The information contained within this book was obtained by the authors from
reliable sources. However, while every effort has been made to ensure its
accuracy, no responsibility for loss, damage or injury occasioned to any person
acting or refraining from action as a result of information contained herein can
be accepted by the publisher or the authors.

PasTest Revision Books and Intensive Courses

*PasTest has been established in the field of undergraduate and
postgraduate medical education since 1972, providing revision books and
intensive study courses for doctors preparing for their professional
examinations. Books and courses are available for:*

MRCGP, MRCP Parts 1 and 2, MRCPCH Parts 1 and 2, MRCS, MRCOG Parts 1
and 2, DRCOG, DCH, FRCA, Dentistry

For further details contact:

**PasTest Ltd, Freepost, Knutsford, Cheshire, WA16 7BR
Tel: 01565 752000   Fax: 01565 650264
www.pastest.co.uk   enquiries@pastest.co.uk**

Cover photo of Amber Hosie-Martin, age 3 months, reproduced with kind
permission of the parents

Typeset by Saxon Graphics Ltd, Derby
Printed and bound in the UK by CPI Antony Rowe

Contents

Contributors

Jim Baird BM MRCPCH
SpR in Paediatric Endocrinology, Paediatric Medical Unit, Southampton General Hospital, Southampton *(Endocrinology)*

R Mark Beattie BSc MBBS FRCPCH MRCP
Consultant Paediatric Gastroenterologist, Paediatric Medical Unit, Southampton General Hospital, Southampton *(Gastroenterology and Nutrition)*

Natalie L E Canham MBChB BA (Hons) MRCP (Paeds)
Consultant in Clinical Genetics, North West Thames Regional Genetics Service, Northwick Park Hospital, Harrow, Middlesex *(Genetics)*

Michael L Capra MBBCh DCH Dip Obs MRCP MMedSci (Clinical education)
Consultant Paediatric Oncologist, Our Lady's Children's Hospital, Dublin *(Clinical Pharmacology; Haematology and Oncology)*

Mike Champion BSc MBBS MRCP FRCPCH
Consultant in Paediatric Inherited Metabolic Disease, Evelina Children's Hospital, Guy's and St Thomas' NHS Foundation Trust, London *(Metabolic Medicine; Ophthalmology)*

Andrew Clark MBBS MRCP MD
Consultant in Paediatric Allergy, Addenbrookes Hospital, Cambridge University Hospitals NHS Foundation Trust, Cambridge *(Respiratory Medicine)*

Serena Cottrell MBBS BSc (Hons) MMedSci MRCPI FRCPCH
Consultant Paediatrician and Lead for Resuscitation Service, Department of Paediatrics, Southampton General Hospital, Southampton *(Emergency Medicine)*

Justin Davies MD FRCPCH MRCP
Consultant Paediatric Endocrinologist, Paediatric Medical Unit, Southampton General Hospital, Southampton *(Endocrinology)*

Jane C Davies MB ChB MRCP MRCPCH MD
Senior Lecturer in Gene Therapy, The Department of Gene Therapy, NHLI, Imperial College, Emmanuel Kaye Building, London *(Respiratory Medicine)*

Anil Dhawan MBBS MD FRCPCH
Professor of Paediatric Hepatology, Paediatric Liver Centre, King's College Hospital, Denmark Hill, London *(Hepatology)*

Katy Fidler BSc MBBS MRCPCH PhD
Consultant in General Paediatrics and Paediatric Infectious Diseases, Royal Alexandra Children's Hospital, Brighton *(Infectious Diseases)*

Grenville F Fox MBChB MRCP FRCPCH
Consultant Neonatologist and Clinical Director, Children's Services and Genetics, Evelina Children's Hospital Neonatal Unit, Guy's and St Thomas' NHS Foundation Trust, London *(Neonatology)*

Helen M Goodyear MBChB FRCP FRCPCH MD MMEd
Consultant Paediatrician and Associate Postgraduate Dean, Department of Child Health, Birmingham Heartlands Hospital, Bordesley Green East, Birmingham *(Dermatology)*

Juliet C Gray MBBS MA PhD MRCP (Paeds)
Clinical Lecturer in Paediatric Oncology, Southampton General Hospital, Southampton *(Haematology and Oncology)*

Steve Halford MBBS MRCP FCEM
Consultant in Emergency Medicine, Southampton General Hospital, Southampton *(Emergency Medicine)*

James W Hart MBBS BSc (Hons) MRCP (UK) MRCPCH
SpR, Paediatric Medical Unit, Southampton General Hospital, Southampton *(Nephrology)*

Nathan Hasson MBChB FRCPCH
Consultant in Paediatric Rheumatology, The Portland Hospital, London *(Rheumatology)*

Tammy Hedderly MBBS BSc (Hons) MRCPCH
Consultant Paediatric Neurologist, Evelina Children's Hospital and King's College Hospital, London *(Neurology)*

Lara Kitteringham MBChB FRCS (Paed)
Consultant Paediatric Surgeon, Paediatric Surgical Unit, Southampton General Hospital, Southampton *(Paediatric Surgery)*

Vic Larcher MB BChir MA FRCPCH FRCP
Consultant in Paediatrics and Clinical Ethics, Great Ormond Street Hospital,
London *(Ethics, Law and Governance)*

Emma J Lim BMBS MSc MRCP
SpR in Paediatric Infectious Diseases, Department of Paediatric Infectious
Disease, St Mary's Hospital, London *(Infectious Diseases)*

Anne-Marie McMahon BSc MBBS MRCPCH MSc
Consultant in Paediatric Rheumatology, The Leeds Teaching Hospitals NHS
Trust and Sheffield Children's NHS Foundation Trust *(Rheumatology)*

Heather Mitchell BM BCh MA MRCP MRCPCH MRCGP DCH DRCOG
SpR in Paediatric Endocrinology, Department of Paediatric Endocrinology,
University College London Hospitals, London *(Endocrinology)*

Reynella Anne Morenas MBBS BSc MRCPCH
SpR in Paediatric Gastroenterology, Paediatric Medical Unit, Southampton
General Hospital, Southampton *(Gastroenterology and Nutrition)*

Karyn Moshal MBChB MRCP MRCPCH DTMH
Consultant and Lead Clinician in Infectious Diseases, Department of Clinical
Infectious Diseases, Great Ormond Street Hospital for Children NHS
Foundation Trust, Great Ormond Street, London *(Infectious Diseases)*

Joanne Philpot BA MBBS MD MRCPCH
Consultant Paediatrician, Paediatric Department, Wexham Park Hospital,
Slough *(Child Development)*

Stephen Playfor DM
Consultant Paediatric Intensivist, Paediatric Intensive Care Unit, Royal
Manchester Children's Hospital, Manchester *(Emergency Medicine)*

Waseem Qasim BMedSci MRCP MRCPCH PhD
Molecular Immunology, Institute of Child Health, London *(Immunology)*

Nicolas Regamey MD
Assistant Professor, Division of Paediatric Respiratory Medicine, University
Children's Hospital, Bern, Switzerland *(Respiratory Medicine)*

Fiona M Regan MB ChB MRCP
Consultant Paediatrician with a special interest in endocrinology and diabetes, Hillingdon Hospital, Uxbridge, London *Endocrinology*

Christopher Reid MRCP (UK) FRCPCH
Consultant Paediatric Nephrologist, Evelina Children's Hospital, Guy's and St Thomas' NHS Foundation Trust, London *(Nephrology)*

Nancy Tan MBBS MMed (Paeds) MRCPCH (Edin) Dip (FP) Derm (S'pore)
Consultant, Department of Paediatric Medicine, KK Women's and Children's Hospital, Singapore *(Hepatology)*

Stephen Tomlin BPharm MRPharmS ACPP
Consultant Pharmacist, Children's Services, Evelina Children's Hospital, Guy's and St Thomas' NHS Foundation Trust, London *(Clinical Pharmacology)*

Robert M R Tulloh BM BCh MA DM FRCP FRCPCH
Consultant Paediatric Cardiologist, Department of Congenital Heart Disease, Bristol Royal Hospital for Children, Bristol *(Cardiology)*

Angie Wade BSc MSc PhD CStat ILTM
Senior Lecturer in Biostatistics, Centre for Paediatric Epidemiology and Statistics, Institute of Child Health, London *(Statistics)*

Robert A Wheeler MS FRCS LLB (Hons) FRCPCH
Consultant Paediatric and Neonatal Surgeon, Hon. Senior Lecturer in Medical Law, Southampton University Hospitals Trust, Southampton *(Ethics, Law and Governance; Paediatric Surgery)*

Amy Whiting BSc (Hons) MB BS MRCPCH
SpR in Paediatrics, Children's Hospital Oxford, John Radcliffe Hospital, Oxford *(Child Development)*

Louise C Wilson BSc MBChB FRCP
Consultant in Clinical Genetics, Department of Genetics, Institute of Child Health, London *(Genetics)*

Every effort has been made to acknowledge the contributors for this book. However, if there are any omissions this will be rectified at reprint.

Introduction

The new edition of this revision text has been written to accompany *Essential Revision Notes in Paediatrics for MRCPCH* (2nd edition). The questions, in the new examination format, are designed to help facilitate revision for the MRCPCH Part One examination and are also relevant for part one of the DCH examination. The book is split by subject to aid revision planning. Each question has a detailed explanation and so the text can be used as a stand-alone revision aid.

The candidate is advised to consult the RCPCH website for up-to-date information regarding the exam (www.rcpch.ac.uk). The information below is taken from the website and is correct at the time of going to press.

The MRCPCH Part One examination consists of two papers:

Paper One A (Basic Child Health), which focuses on the areas of child health that are relevant to those who will be working with children in their medical careers, not just those entering mainstream hospital-based paediatrics. The areas tested are those conditions likely to be seen in 6 to 12 months of hospital, community or primary care practice.

Paper One B (Extended Paediatrics) focuses on the more complex paediatric problem-solving skills not tested in Paper One A, and on the scientific knowledge underpinning paediatrics.

Candidates for MRCPCH must successfully complete both Paper One A and One B before being allowed to enter MRCPCH Part Two.

Paper One A (Basic Child Health) replaces the previous Diploma in Child Health (DCH) written paper.

The papers consist of:

Multiple true-false questions used to test knowledge when there is an absolute Yes/No answer.

Best of Five questions used to test judgement and experience. A simple statement or short clinical scenario leads into five options. All could be possible but only one is completely or the most correct. The candidate has to choose the best option.

Extended matching questions (EMQs) are used in the same way as Best of Five questions. In this case a list of 6–12 possible answers is offered with two or three statements or clinical scenarios. The candidate chooses the best option from the introductory list. Again, all could be possible but only one is completely or the most correct.

Further details on the make-up of the three types of questions and on the proportion of different types are available on the college website along with downloadable sample papers.

We would like to acknowledge the many authors who have enthusiastically contributed chapters to this book and Kirsten Baxter and Lily Martin at PasTest for their enthusiasm and expertise in helping pull this new edition together.

Finally, we hope the book helps candidates to get through the exam!

Mark Beattie
Mike Champion
August 2009

1. Cardiology

Multiple True–False Questions

1.1 Muscular ventricular septal defects (VSDs)

- [ ] A do not require SBE prophylaxis
- [ ] B usually cause a heart murmur in the first day of life
- [ ] C if large, are closed by catheter procedures in 10% of cases
- [ ] D do not have conduction tissue running on their inferior margin
- [ ] E if large, usually cause heart failure before the child is 4 days old

1.2 Scimitar syndrome

- [ ] A is usually associated with a hypoplastic left lung
- [ ] B can be palliated by coil occlusion in the cardiac catheter laboratory
- [ ] C will show dextrocardia on the X-ray as a result of situs inversus
- [ ] D is associated with abnormal pulmonary arterial supply
- [ ] E is usually associated with abnormal radii

1.3 On the first day of life, the following may be found in neonates with congenital heart disease:

- [ ] A a harsh pansystolic murmur with the diagnosis of ventricular septal defect
- [ ] B severe cyanosis in unobstructed total anomalous pulmonary venous connection
- [ ] C a harsh systolic murmur in transposition of the great arteries without associated defect
- [ ] D severe acidosis and poor pulses with hypoplastic left heart syndrome
- [ ] E severe cyanosis and acidosis in a baby with Down syndrome and atrioventricular septal defect

1.4 The following is true of persistent ductus arteriosus:

- [ ] A it is defined as persistence of ductal patency beyond 1 week after the date the baby should have been born
- [ ] B on auscultation, a continuous murmur in the right infraclavicular area is heard
- [ ] C it may present as heart failure with poor peripheral pulses
- [ ] D closure is usually undertaken in the catheter laboratory with coil or device at 1 year
- [ ] E if it is large, surgical ligation is recommended at 1–3 months

1.5 The following statements about transposition of the great arteries are true:

☐ A   there is an association with coarctation of the aorta

☐ B   arterial switch is the operation of choice, undertaken before 2 weeks

☐ C   the condition is detected antenatally in 50% of cases

☐ D   presentation can occur upon closure of the ductus arteriosus

☐ E   the arrangement of the coronary arteries is a major factor in determining the success of the surgical repair

1.6 The following is true of Eisenmenger syndrome:

☐ A   affected children are typically teenagers

☐ B   it can be seen in children with Down syndrome

☐ C   it is usually secondary to an untreated ventricular septal defect or atrioventricular septal defect

☐ D   the pulmonary component of the second heart sound is quiet on auscultation

☐ E   the ECG shows left ventricular hypertrophy

Best of Five Questions

1.7 You are asked to review an ECG of a baby on the intensive care unit. The baby was well at birth, but soon became unwell and cyanosed. There was no heart murmur. ECG findings reveal a superior axis, absent right ventricular voltages, and a large P wave. What is the MOST likely diagnosis?

☐ A   Complete atrioventricular septal defect

☐ B   Tricuspid atresia

☐ C   Critical pulmonary stenosis

☐ D   Transposition of the great arteries

☐ E   Total anomalous pulmonary venous connection (TAPVC)

1.8 You are asked to see in clinic a 6-year-old girl with a diagnosis of right atrial isomerism. Which one of the following features would you expect her to have?

☐ A   Asplenia and a midline liver

☐ B   Polysplenia

☐ C   Two functional left lungs

☐ D   T-cell deficiency

☐ E   Trisomy 21

1.9 You are asked to review a child on the ward who is known to have short stature and renal abnormalities. On examination, she has micrognathia and an ejection systolic murmur at the upper left sternal edge. Her notes show that she has recently seen an ophthalmologist. What is the MOST likely underlying diagnosis?

- ☐ A Williams syndrome
- ☐ B DiGeorge syndrome
- ☐ C Alagille syndrome
- ☐ D Noonan syndrome
- ☐ E Left atrial isomerism

1.10 A 1-day-old baby who is otherwise asymptomatic presents with a loud harsh heart murmur at the left sternal edge. There are no features of heart failure present, the oxygen saturations are normal, and the ECG performed by the resident speciality registrar is reported to be normal. What is the MOST likely diagnosis in this case?

- ☐ A Atrial septal defect
- ☐ B Small muscular ventricular septal defect
- ☐ C Large muscular ventricular septal defect
- ☐ D Pulmonary stenosis
- ☐ E Persistent ductus arteriosus

1.11 A newborn baby presents cyanosed and unwell with a heart murmur at the left sternal edge. The chest X-ray shows massive cardiomegaly with a dilated right atrium and reduced pulmonary vascular markings. You are informed that the baby's mother has a history of bipolar depression and that she had been taking lithium during pregnancy. What is the MOST likely diagnosis?

- ☐ A Transposition of the great arteries
- ☐ B Tetralogy of Fallot
- ☐ C Tricuspid atresia
- ☐ D Ebstein anomaly
- ☐ E Pulmonary atresia, ventricular septal defect and collaterals

1.12 A 2-year-old boy presents with a murmur, heard in both systole and diastole at the upper sternal edge, which disappears on lying down. Physical examination is otherwise normal. He is a well, asymptomatic child and there are no signs of cardiac failure. You are told that his second cousin had a small ventricular septal defect, which closed spontaneously, and that his uncle had a heart attack aged 45. What do you consider to be the BEST management plan?

- ☐ A   Refer for echocardiography and specialist opinion from a consultant paediatric cardiologist
- ☐ B   Perform an ECG, chest X-ray and oxygen saturations, and then refer for echocardiography
- ☐ C   Refer for genetic counselling and, possibly, gene-mapping studies
- ☐ D   Reassure them that the murmur is innocent
- ☐ E   Say that you suspect the murmur is caused by a persistent arterial duct, which should be coil-occluded to avoid the development of heart failure in the future

1.13 You are asked to review a 4-month-old girl in clinic. Her ECG shows a short P–R interval and giant QRS complexes. Echocardiography reveals evidence of hypertrophic cardiomyopathy. What is the MOST likely diagnosis?

- ☐ A   Pompe disease
- ☐ B   Lown–Ganong–Levine syndrome
- ☐ C   Hurler syndrome
- ☐ D   Noonan syndrome
- ☐ E   Wolff–Parkinson–White syndrome

Extended Matching Questions

1.14 Theme: Surgical procedures in paediatric cardiology

A   Arterial switch procedure
B   Hemi-Fontan
C   Fontan
D   Norwood
E   Rastelli
F   Blalock–Taussig shunt
G   Pulmonary artery (PA) band
H   Ductus arteriosus ligation
I   Coarctation of the aorta repair

From the list above, choose the most appropriate procedure for the children in the scenarios below. Each option may be used once, more than once, or not at all.

☐ 1. A 4-day-old baby who presented with absent femoral and brachial pulses, no heart murmur, and severe acidosis. ECG had revealed absent left ventricular forces.

☐ 2. A 3-year-old child with complex cardiac problems, which were not suitable for repair, including two separate ventricles. He had undergone a previous heart operation at the age of 7 months and had oxygen saturations of 80–85%. His cardiologist felt that he required a further operation, as there was insufficient blood flow to the lungs, causing exercise limitation.

☐ 3. A severely cyanosed baby with tetralogy of Fallot and a loud heart murmur at the upper left sternal edge, and a recent history of severe spells of cyanosis.

1.15 Theme: The sick newborn infant

A   Pulmonary atresia
B   Tetralogy of Fallot
C   Coarctation of the aorta
D   Hypoplastic left heart syndrome
E   Transposition of the great arteries
F   Interrupted aortic arch
G   Obstructed total anomalous pulmonary venous connection
H   Critical aortic stenosis
I   Ebstein anomaly

Choose the most likely diagnosis from the histories and findings detailed below. Each option may be used once, more than once, or not at all.

☐ 1. A 6-day-old baby presents cyanosed, with a severe metabolic acidosis. On examination, there is a large liver but no audible heart murmur. ECG and chest X-ray were both reported to be normal.

☐ 2. A breathless baby with a cleft palate, absent left brachial and femoral pulses, and a normal ECG.

☐ 3. A very unwell baby, with a loud heart murmur, a superior axis on the ECG, and reduced pulmonary vascular markings on the chest X-ray.

MT–F Answers

1.1   Muscular ventricular septal defects (VSDs): D

Ventricular septal defects are the most common form of congenital heart disease, comprising 30% of the total number of cases. Muscular VSDs occur in the muscular part of the ventricular septum. Subacute bacterial endocarditis (SBE) prophylaxis is no longer indicated, now only being required in rare and specific cases. The pulmonary resistance is high at birth, and hence there is little shunt between the two ventricles and therefore no audible murmur in the first 24 hours. Only 25% of VSDs require cardiac surgery, and this is usually performed when the child is 3–5 months of age. Very few patients have interventional catheter closure, usually for smaller defects and at a later age. The conduction tissue is located inferiorly in a perimembranous septal defect, which means that surgeons need to avoid that area when suturing a patch in place to close the defect. If the VSD is large, patients present with symptoms of heart failure after the first week of life and at that age have a right ventricular heave, a soft systolic murmur accompanied by an apical mid-diastolic murmur, and a loud pulmonary second heart sound on examination.

1.2   Scimitar syndrome: B D

Scimitar syndrome is a form of anomalous pulmonary venous drainage in which the veins from the lower right lung drain into the inferior vena cava. The right lung itself is hypoplastic, and there is an associated dextrocardia due to the heart moving over to the right side of the chest, but with normal situs. Situs is the orientation of the organs, situs solitus being normal, and situs inversus being mirror image. The arterial supply to the lung is from branches of the descending aorta. The right upper lobe pulmonary vein draining into the inferior vena cava may be seen as a vertical line on a chest X-ray and is known as the 'scimitar sign'. There may be an atrial septal defect, and children can suffer with recurrent chest infections, which may require right lower lobectomy.

1.3   Congenital heart disease on the first day of life: D E

Babies presenting with left-to-right shunt will have no murmur or symptoms on the first day of life, because the pulmonary vascular resistance has yet to fall. Similarly, any common mixing disease, such as atrioventricular septal defect, can present with severe cyanosis on the first day of life, with high pulmonary vascular resistance, before breathlessness and heart failure develop at 1 week of age or more. All the obstructed left heart lesions, such as coarctation of the aorta and hypoplastic left heart syndrome, tend to present with acidosis and weak pulses in the first few days of life.

1.4   Persistent ductus arteriosus: D E

There is abnormal persistence of the ductus arteriosus beyond 1 month after the date the baby should have been born. Those children affected are usually asymptomatic and rarely develop heart failure. On auscultation, a continuous 'machinery' or systolic murmur at the left infraclavicular area is heard. The murmur is initially systolic but, as the pulmonary vascular resistance falls, it becomes continuous in nature because there is a continual run-off of blood from the aorta to the pulmonary artery (as the pressure in the aorta is greater than in the pulmonary artery throughout the cardiac cycle). Other clinical features include bounding pulses and wide pulse pressure. If the duct is large, chest radiography can demonstrate cardiomegaly and pulmonary plethora. Management is usually by closure in the cardiac catheter laboratory with a coil or device when the infant is 1 year of age. However, if the duct is large, surgical ligation can be undertaken when the infant is aged 1–3 months. The presence of a ductus arteriosus in a pre-term baby is not congenital heart disease, but these children have a higher incidence of persistent ductus arteriosus.

1.5   Transposition of the great arteries: A B D E

In this condition, the aorta usually arises anteriorly from the right ventricle and the pulmonary artery arises posteriorly from the left ventricle. Deoxygenated blood is therefore returned to the body, while oxygenated blood goes back to the lungs. If these two parallel circuits were completely separate, the condition would be incompatible with life. These children have high pulmonary blood flow and are very cyanosed, unless there is an atrial septal defect, a ductus arteriosus, or a ventricular septal defect, allowing mixing of the two circulations. Babies become cyanosed when the duct closes, thus reducing the mixing between the systemic and pulmonary circulations, but there is usually no murmur. Transposition of the great arteries may be associated with ventricular septal defect, coarctation of the aorta or pulmonary stenosis. Management is to resuscitate the baby, followed by a balloon atrial septostomy (preferably via the umbilical vein) at a cardiac centre in about 20% of cases. In the sick, cyanosed newborn baby, a continuous intravenous infusion of prostaglandin E_1 or E_2 should be commenced to keep the duct open. Definitive repair in the form of the arterial switch operation will usually be undertaken before the baby is 2 weeks of age.

1.6   Eisenmenger syndrome: A B C

Eisenmenger syndrome was first described in 1897, and occurs secondary to a large left-to-right shunt (usually a ventricular septal defect or atrioventricular septal defect) in which the pulmonary hypertension leads to pulmonary vascular disease (increased resistance over many years). Eventually, the flow through the defect is reversed (right-to-left) so the child becomes blue, typically at 10–15 years of age. There is not usually a significant heart murmur. Eventually, they develop right heart failure. The ECG shows right ventricular hypertrophy and strain pattern, with peaked P waves indicating right atrial hypertrophy. Management is largely supportive, as surgical closure is not possible when there is a right-to-left shunt. They may be commenced on sildenafil or an endothelin-receptor antagonist on the advice of a specialist in pulmonary hypertension.

Best of Five Answers

1.7   B: Tricuspid atresia

Tricuspid atresia is the condition in which there is no tricuspid valve and usually the right ventricle is very small. There is right-to-left shunt at atrial level, as the blood cannot pass into the right ventricle. Babies become very cyanosed when the ductus arteriosus closes if they are duct-dependent, and they usually have no heart murmur. Management options include a Blalock–Taussig shunt if the child is very blue, a pulmonary artery (PA) band if they are in heart failure, a hemi-Fontan procedure after they reach 6 months of age, and a Fontan procedure at 3–5 years of age. The ECG shows a superior axis, as the atrioventricular junction is located inferiorly, the P waves are large as a result of right atrial hypertension, and there is a small right ventricle, reducing the forces visible on the ECG.

1.8   A: Asplenia and a midline liver

Right atrial isomerism is a multifactorial genetic defect. Right atrial isomerism is associated with asplenia, small-bowel malrotation, and complex heart disease with abnormalities of connection, in which the pulmonary veins always connect abnormally because there is no morphological left atrium with which to connect. In left atrial isomerism, there is polysplenia, small-bowel malrotation (less common than in right atrial isomerism), two left lungs and complex heart disease.

1.9   C: Alagille syndrome

Alagille syndrome is a genetic defect of the *JAG-1* gene in 70% of cases. Features include peripheral pulmonary artery stenosis, a prominent forehead, wide-apart eyes, small chin, butterfly vertebrae, intrahepatic biliary hypoplasia, embryotoxon (slit lamp for cornea), and renal and growth abnormalities. Posterior embryotoxon occurs when there is a prominent Schwalbe's line visible just inside the temporal limbus. It occurs in approximately 15% of normal eyes and is visible through a clear cornea as a sharply defined, concentric white line or opacity anterior to the limbus. Williams syndrome is due to a 1.5-Mb deletion on chromosome 7 and leads to typical facial features, behavioural abnormalities and cardiac features of supravalvar aortic stenosis and branch pulmonary artery stenosis. DiGeorge syndrome is associated with conotruncal defects (tetralogy of Fallot, common arterial trunk and interrupted aortic arch), typical facial features, cleft palate, absent thymus and absent parathyroids. Noonan syndrome is associated with mutations in *PTPN11*, *SOS1*, *KRAS* or *RAF1* genes, with cardiac features of hypertrophic cardiomyopathy, atrial septal defect, pulmonary stenosis and pulmonary hypertension.

1.10 D: Pulmonary stenosis

Those children with left-to-right shunts have no signs or symptoms on the first day of life. However, those with outflow obstruction have a murmur from birth. Pulmonary stenosis usually causes no cyanosis, and all neonates have a dominant right ventricle, thus revealing no evidence of right ventricular hypertrophy.

1.11 D: Ebstein anomaly

Ebstein anomaly is signified by an abnormal and regurgitant tricuspid valve, which is set further down into the right ventricle than normal. The affected child will be cyanosed at birth, with a pansystolic murmur of tricuspid regurgitation at the lower sternal edge. This congenital heart condition has been associated with maternal ingestion of lithium.

1.12 D: Reassure them that the murmur is innocent

This is typical of a venous hum, an innocent heart murmur. It may be easy to hear the venous blood flow returning to the heart, especially at the upper sternal edge. This characteristically occurs in both systole and diastole, and disappears when the child lies flat. Innocent murmurs are the most common murmurs heard in children, occurring in up to 50% of normal children. They are often discovered in children with a co-existing infection or with anaemia.

Innocent murmurs all relate to a structurally normal heart and it is clearly important to reassure the parents that their child's heart is normal. Types of innocent murmur include those caused by increased flow across the branch pulmonary artery, Still's murmur, and venous hums. The murmur should be soft (no thrill), systolic (diastolic murmurs are not innocent) and short, never pansystolic. The child is always asymptomatic. The murmur may change with posture, as in venous hums.

1.13 A: Pompe disease

Pompe disease is a glycogen storage disorder that can affect the heart. It results in an autosomal recessive hypertrophic cardiomyopathy, and is rare. Glycogen accumulates in skeletal muscle, the tongue and diaphragm, and the liver. The heart enlarges as glycogen is deposited in the ventricular muscle. It is a progressive disease. The ECG reveals a short P–R interval with giant QRS complexes. Chest radiography shows an enlarged heart and often congested lung fields. Treatment is largely supportive.

EMQ Answers

1.14 Surgical procedures in paediatric cardiology

1. D: Norwood procedure

The Norwood procedure is used to palliate hypoplastic left heart syndrome. It is performed when the infant is aged 3–5 days. The right ventricle is intended to pump blood to the body, so the pulmonary artery is sewn onto the aorta. The atrial septum is excised so that pulmonary venous blood can return to the right ventricle and, to ensure adequate pulmonary blood flow, either a Blalock–Taussig shunt is inserted or a conduit is constructed from the right ventricle to the pulmonary arteries. As there is a small left ventricle, there is little voltage from this chamber.

2. C: Fontan procedure

The Fontan operation is a palliative procedure and is usually performed when the patient is 3–5 years of age. A channel is inserted to drain blood from the inferior vena cava to the right pulmonary artery. Blue deoxygenated blood then flows directly to the lungs and bypasses the heart. The oxygenated blood comes back from the lungs and is pumped by the ventricle to the body.

3. F: Blalock–Taussig shunt

A Blalock–Taussig systemic-to-pulmonary shunt will increase pulmonary blood flow in the severely cyanosed baby with tetralogy of Fallot and a recent history of severe spells of cyanosis. Most of these children go on to have elective surgical repair at 6–9 months to close the ventricular septal defect and widen the right ventricular outflow tract.

1.15 The sick newborn infant

1. G: Obstructed total anomalous pulmonary venous connection

In total anomalous pulmonary venous connection, the pulmonary veins do not make the normal connection with the left atrium. Instead, they can drain upwards to the innominate vein, to the liver or to the coronary sinus. If the connection becomes obstructed, the baby will present at 1–7 days of life with cyanosis, acidosis, breathlessness, collapse, and signs of right heart failure, and will require emergency resuscitation, ventilation and surgery.

2. F: Interrupted aortic arch

Interrupted aortic arch can occur at any site from the innominate artery as far as distal to the left subclavian artery. It is a duct-dependent condition and is associated with DiGeorge syndrome. In DiGeorge syndrome, there is cardiac disease, 22q11.2 gene deletion, absent thymus, absent parathyroids, abnormal facies, and cleft palate. Affected babies usually present with absent left brachial and femoral pulses, and signs of heart failure when the ductus arteriosus closes.

3. I: Ebstein anomaly

In Ebstein anomaly, the tricuspid valve is abnormal: the posterior leaflet of the tricuspid valve originates within the right ventricular cavity, which is thus 'atrialised'. A huge right atrium results from the inability of the right ventricle to pump blood forward into the pulmonary artery and therefore sometimes a palliative Blalock–Taussig shunt has to be inserted. Affected babies present with a loud heart murmur (tricuspid regurgitation), a superior axis on the ECG, and reduced pulmonary vascular markings on chest X-ray, with an enlarged cardiac silhouette.

2. Child Development, Child Psychiatry and Community Paediatrics

Multiple True–False Questions

2.1   Characteristics of fragile X syndrome include:
- [ ] A   micro-orchidism in postpubertal males
- [ ] B   male preponderance
- [ ] C   typical facial features of micrognathia and long facies
- [ ] D   poor eye contact and social impairment
- [ ] E   absence of learning disability in all females

2.2   Regarding gross motor development and posture,
- [ ] A   a 6-week-old lying in the supine position will show extension at the elbows, hips and knees
- [ ] B   a 2-month-old held in ventral suspension will not be able to hold his head in line with his body
- [ ] C   a 3-month-old in the prone position will lift his head and upper chest, supported by his forearms
- [ ] D   a 6-month-old would be expected to roll over
- [ ] E   a 6-month-old would be expected to sit unsupported and reach out for nearby objects

2.3   A typical 1-year-old is able to
- [ ] A   feed himself with a biscuit
- [ ] B   use the index finger to point to what he wants
- [ ] C   pick up small crumbs with the thumb and index finger
- [ ] D   look for toys he has dropped
- [ ] E   bang together two objects in the midline

2.4   Criteria for a successful screening test include:
- [ ] A   the condition is important and rare
- [ ] B   an identified and available treatment pathway
- [ ] C   moderate numbers of true positives (sensitivity)
- [ ] D   early intervention to be as effective as late intervention at improving outcome
- [ ] E   acceptability to the patient and family

2.5 A typical 5-month-old should display the following visually directed behaviours:

☐ A grasp a small-sized object
☐ B follow large objects to the midline
☐ C look at a face
☐ D follow large objects beyond the midline
☐ E follow large objects over 180°

2.6 Medical complications of bulimia nervosa include:

☐ A fluid and electrolyte imbalance
☐ B thyroid gland enlargement
☐ C peri-oral callus formation
☐ D enamel erosion of the teeth
☐ E oesophagitis

Best of Five Questions

2.7 A 7-year-old girl attends the outpatient clinic with a history of day- and night-time wetting. She has never been fully continent of urine; she passes small amounts of urine regularly throughout the day, becoming more frequent in the afternoon. Her mother's pregnancy and the girl's delivery had been uneventful. The girl has not had any significant illnesses, and is developmentally normal. She lives with her parents and two older siblings. She says she is happy at home and at school. She is progressing well with her school work. She doesn't enjoy sports at school and often misses physical education lessons. She appears to be embarrassed by her problem, and her parents seem appropriately concerned. On examination she looks well. Her general examination and neurological examination are normal. Her spine is normal. There is no palpable bladder or kidneys. Her urine dip is negative for leukocytes and nitrites. Which of the following is the MOST likely diagnosis?

☐ A Ectopic ureter
☐ B Neurogenic bladder
☐ C Urinary tract infection
☐ D Delayed maturation of urethral sphincter control
☐ E Detrusor instability

2.8 An 8-year-old girl attends the outpatients department with a 3-month history of non-attendance at school. She says little in the clinic room. Parents describe how she had seemed happy at school at the end of the previous term, and her teacher had been very happy with her academic progress and behaviour in school. She is the younger of two children and lives with both her parents. The parents do not report any difficulties at home. They have both worked full-time since she was a baby. Her child-minder has been taking her to school with her sister, but when they arrive at the school gate she becomes distressed and will not enter the playground. Her mother's pregnancy and the girl's delivery had been uneventful. Her general health is fine. Developmentally, she appears to be age-appropriate. She has not had her full schedule of immunisations because her parents did not want her to have her MMR vaccine at the pre-school vaccinations. Her examination is unremarkable. Which of the following is the MOST likely cause of her school non-attendance?

☐ A Truancy
☐ B School phobia
☐ C Conduct disorder
☐ D Depression
☐ E Bullying

2.9 A 3-year-old boy is referred to the outpatient department with concerns about his development. The pregnancy and neonatal history were uneventful, and he has had no serious illnesses. He has always been slow in his development. His mother also had mild learning difficulties, and needed extra help in school. On assessment, he can walk but cannot jump. He has poor eye contact, has no clear words, and can not identify parts of his body. He is unable to copy a horizontal line, and is still in nappies. Examination is very difficult, because he becomes very distressed and demonstrates hand flapping. His head circumference is on the 90th centile. Which of the following is the MOST useful investigation?

☐ A Thyroid studies
☐ B Magnetic resonance imaging (MRI) brain scan
☐ C Urinary organic acids
☐ D Genetic studies
☐ E Electroencephalogram (EEG)

2.10 A 3-year-old boy is referred to the outpatient department with concerns about speech and language development. The pregnancy and neonatal history were uneventful and he has had no serious illnesses. At 15 months he had five clear words that he has since stopped using. He enjoys puzzles, is able to feed using a spoon and fork, and can dress himself with help. There has been difficulty settling him into nursery. He becomes very distressed and runs around being disruptive and sometimes physically aggressive towards other children. On assessment he is very difficult to settle and tries to escape from the room. He does not demonstrate any clear words or understanding of simple commands and refuses to engage in any activities. Which of the following is the MOST likely diagnosis?

- [ ] A Attention deficit disorder
- [ ] B Specific speech and language delay
- [ ] C Autistic spectrum disorder
- [ ] D Deafness
- [ ] E Global developmental delay

2.11 A 14-year-old girl is seen in clinic with a history of a severe sore throat and fever 4 months previously. Since then she has had headaches, generalised muscle pain, tiredness, and poor concentration of increasing severity. For the past 2 months she has been unable to attend school because of her muscle pain and lethargy, and her sleep pattern has become disturbed. She finds it very difficult to fall asleep at night, and then has difficulty getting up in the morning. On examination she has mild lymphadenopathy and looks pale. Her weight is continuing along the 25th centile. Examination is otherwise unremarkable, except for the marked muscle pain she experiences on movement of her limbs. Which of the following is the MOST likely diagnosis?

- [ ] A Depression
- [ ] B Chronic fatigue syndrome
- [ ] C Hypothyroidism
- [ ] D Crohn's disease
- [ ] E Anorexia nervosa

2.12 A 13-year-old girl is seen in clinic with a history of weight loss over the previous 6 months. Her weight has gone from the 75th to the 3rd centile and her height has continued along the 50th. Apart from her periods, which have stopped, her general health has been fine. She is in the county's gymnastic squad, but over the past 2 months she has missed training sessions. Her examination is unremarkable. Which of the following is the MOST likely diagnosis?

- [ ] A Depression
- [ ] B Chronic fatigue syndrome
- [ ] C Hyperthyroidism
- [ ] D Crohn's disease
- [ ] E Anorexia nervosa

2.13 A 15-month-old child is seen in clinic with a 3-month history of collapsing. The episodes occur when he has been hurt. He suddenly looks very pale, loses consciousness, and falls to the floor. He then appears to stiffen, and has some clonic movements of his arms and legs before quickly recovering. Examination is unremarkable. Which of the following is the MOST likely diagnosis?

- [ ] A Prolonged QT syndrome
- [ ] B Reflex anoxic seizures
- [ ] C Complex partial epilepsy
- [ ] D Tonic–clonic seizures
- [ ] E Myoclonic seizures

Extended Matching Questions

2.14 Theme: Speech delay

A Electroencephalogram (EEG)
B Urine organic acids
C Creatine kinase
D Brain magnetic resonance imaging (MRI)
E Hearing assessment
F Lactate
G Genetic studies for fragile X
H Electrocardiogram (ECG)
I Ammonia

For each patient below, select the most appropriate investigation from those listed above. Each option may be used once, more than once, or not at all.

☐ 1. A 3-year-old boy presents with loss of language skills. Speech development appeared to be normal until his 3rd birthday, following which he has become progressively more aphasic.

☐ 2. A 3-year-old boy presents with delay in expressive speech and comprehension. Questioning reveals that he walked at 21 months and had his first clear word at 2 years. His eye contact is normal, but it is difficult to keep him on task. On developmental assessment, he can copy vertical lines, but not a circle. He can identify animals in a book, and one colour. Expressively, he is not putting two words together. He is still wearing nappies.

☐ 3. A 3-year-old boy presents with delay in expressive speech and comprehension. On questioning, he walked at 24 months and had his first clear word at 2 years. His eye contact is poor, and it is very difficult to keep him on task. On developmental assessment, he can scribble, but prefers fiddling with the crayons and chewing them. He cannot point to parts of his body, and grunts in response to questions. No clear words are demonstrated. He is still wearing nappies. He has an uncle, now aged 28, who is known to have developmental delay and was very slow to walk.

2.15 Theme: Children Act

A   Place of Safety Order
B   Care Order
C   Wardship
D   Child Assessment Order
E   Supervision Order
F   Police Protection Order
G   Emergency Protection Order (EPO)
H   Statementing Order

Identify the following orders of the Children Act 1989 below from those listed above. Each option may be used once, more than once, or not at all.

☐   1. This order lasts for a maximum of 8 days, with a possibility of extension for a further 7 days. This order may be granted by the court if there is reason to believe that a child may be harmed if not removed from their present accommodation.

☐   2. This order confers parental responsibility on the social services (in addition to that of the parents), and usually involves removal from home. It may be applied for in cases of non-accidental injury in which enquires will take some time, and when the child is not regarded as being safe at home.

☐   3. This order may be used if there is a situation of persistent but non-urgent suspicion of risk. It overrides the objections of a parent to whatever examination or assessment is needed to see whether the child is at significant risk of harm. This order lasts up to 7 days.

MT−F Answers

2.1   Characteristics of fragile X syndrome: B D

Fragile X syndrome is an X-linked condition affecting 1 in 4000 males and is characterised by learning disability. It was first recognised following an observation that there were many more males than females with learning disability. The fragile X chromosome marker is a breakage gap at the distal q arm of the X chromosome. At this site, a CGG triplet expansion inactivates distal genes. Fragile X syndrome causes moderate to severe learning disability in males, and can cause learning disability in carrier females. It is characterised by a long face, prominent ears and jaw, and macro-orchidism in postpubertal males. Behavioural characteristics include social impairment, poor attention, and difficulty in making and sustaining eye contact.

2.2   Gross motor development and posture: C D

At 6 weeks, a baby placed in the supine position will classically show a flexed posture at the elbows, hips and knees. An extended posture may indicate cerebral palsy. A 6-week-old held in ventral suspension will be expected to be able to hold his head in line with his body. At 3 months, a baby placed face-down should be able to lift their head and upper chest, supported by their forearms. Rolling over is usually achieved by 6 months. It is not until 9 months that a baby would be expected to sit totally unsupported while reaching out to grasp objects.

2.3   Typical 1-year-old: A C D E

At 9 months of age a child will look for toys they have dropped and will have developed a mature grip between the thumb and index finger. By 1 year of age, they can use this pincer grip to pick up small crumbs. At 1 year, a child is expected to be able to bang together two objects in the midline and to feed himself a biscuit. By 15 months a child should be able to point to what he wants, using his index finger.

2.4   Criteria for a successful screening test: B E

Successful screening tests require the **condition** to be important, with a well-understood natural history and epidemiology. The **test** itself should be cost-effective, acceptable to the patient and family, and sensitive (high number of true positives) and specific (low number of false negatives); the pathway for further diagnostic evaluation should have been agreed. The **treatment** pathway should be clearly understood, available, evidence-based, and should provide an early intervention that improves outcome. The **screening programme** should be effective at reducing mortality and morbidity, cost-effective, and acceptable to the community as a whole. It will require continuing quality assurance and audit.

2.5　Visually directed behaviours: B C D E

In the first year, visually directed behaviours develop in response to normal visual system maturation. It is normal for an infant to look at a face before 6 weeks, follow large objects to the midline from 2 weeks to 2 months, and beyond the midline at 2–3 months of age. Following large objects over 180° occurs between 3 and 5 months. Grasping small objects is a later skill, developed from 9 months of age. Visually directed behaviours are crude measures of the visual system, but do highlight more severe visual impairments.

2.6　Medical complications of bulimia nervosa: A D E

The repetitive binge eating and vomiting in bulimia nervosa can result in fluid and electrolyte imbalance. Excessive use of laxatives and diuretics can also exacerbate metabolic disturbance. Salivary gland enlargement and oesophagitis are common. Callus formation on the knuckles occurs from using the hand to induce vomiting. Enamel erosion occurs as a result of the acidity of regurgitated stomach contents. Thyroid gland enlargement is not characteristic of bulimia nervosa.

Best of Five Answers

2.7　E: Detrusor instability

Primary daytime enuresis is a lack of attainment of bladder control in the daytime and is often accompanied by night-time incontinence of urine. An organic aetiology is present in fewer than 5% of cases. In the majority of cases, there is a delay in the maturation of normal urethral sphincter control mechanisms. There are often co-existent psychological or developmental problems. In this patient an ectopic ureter is unlikely, as incontinence would be worse in the morning from pooling of the urine in the bladder overnight. Normal neurology, spine, and a non-distended bladder make neurogenic bladder unlikely. Urinary tract infection in light of a negative urine dip for leukocytes and nitrites is unlikely, although in this case a clean-catch urine sample should be sent for microscopy, culture and sensitivity. Delayed maturation of sphincter control is possible, although there seem to be no psychological, developmental, or behavioural problems, and no obvious family stressors. Detrusor instability is a result of intermittent contraction of the detrusor muscle during the filling and storage stage of the bladder when it should be relaxed, producing urine leakage and urge incontinence. It is more common in girls, and produces minor degrees of wetness that becomes worse in the afternoon. Treatment involves regular bladder emptying and positive reinforcement. Oxybutynin therapy has been used to stabilise the detrusor muscle.

2.8   B: School phobia

Non-attendance at school is a complex problem. There are three main types of school non-attendance:

- Children who have a good reason not to attend, for example because of bullying or an inability to cope with school work.
- The so-called neurotic disorders of school refusal. These can result from separation anxiety (for example, fear of being away from parents or carers) or school phobia (a fear of school). School refusal is more common in children of primary school age who come from stable family backgrounds. They tend to be the only or youngest child, and are usually doing very well academically. In this girl, school phobia would be the most likely diagnosis, as the fear and difficulty arise on her arrival at school, as opposed to on separation from the parents.
- Truancy, a conduct disorder that is more common in children of secondary school age. They tend to exhibit antisocial behaviours both at home and in school, and are generally lower achievers. Children who truant tend to come from larger and more chaotic families with poor adult supervision. School refusal carries a more positive prognosis than school truancy.

2.9   D: Genetic studies

The history tells us that the child is a boy with a mother with learning difficulties. This should always raise concern regarding fragile X and Duchenne muscular dystrophy. The examination reveals a child with significant developmental delay, autistic features and a large head, all in keeping with a diagnosis of fragile X. The other investigations are reasonable in a child with developmental delay, but in this individual are less likely to provide a diagnosis.

2.10 C: Autistic spectrum disorder

From the history, some of this child's development is age-appropriate, excluding global developmental delay. The history and his behaviour in clinic make specific speech and language delay and deafness unlikely. Attention deficit disorder is a possibility, but it would not explain his regression of language at around 15 months of age and the severe delay in speech and language since. It is also unusual to make a diagnosis of attention deficit disorder in such a young child. Autistic spectrum disorder would explain all the findings and is the most likely diagnosis.

2.11 B: Chronic fatigue syndrome

The lack of weight loss excludes anorexia nervosa and makes Crohn's disease unlikely. If hypothyroidism was severe enough to cause her to take 2 months off school, her weight would have been expected to increase, thus excluding hypothyroidism as a diagnosis. Depression is a possibility, but the sleep pattern is not typical. Chronic fatigue syndrome often develops after a viral illness. Headaches, generalised muscle pains, poor concentration, and sleep disturbance are all features of the illness. Pallor and mild cervical lymphadenopathy are common. Weight is usually static or can increase slightly as a result of lack of exercise.

2.12 E: Anorexia nervosa

Anorexia is the most likely diagnosis. Crohn's disease is a possibility, but there is no history of any bowel disturbance, despite a dramatic loss in weight. If the patient had hyperthyroidism there should have been some clinical signs on examination, such as tachycardia, sweaty palms or goitre. The history is also not typical of chronic fatigue syndrome.

2.13 B: Reflex anoxic seizures

Although the child appears to stiffen and has some clonic movements of his limbs, complex partial epilepsy, tonic–clonic seizures, and myoclonic seizures are unlikely as the events always occur after a painful stimulus. Reflex anoxic seizures have rapid onset, and the child looks pale, becomes bradycardic, and sometimes asystolic; there is a brief convulsion and a quick recovery. Tiredness and pallor may persist for a short time following a seizure. Reflex anoxic seizures are also known as **pallid** breath-holding spells. **Cyanotic** breath-holding spells occur in children younger than 3 years and involve a prolonged expiratory apnoea and cerebral anoxia. The child becomes cyanotic, collapses, and has brief tonic–clonic movements. This condition tends to be self-limiting.

EMQ Answers

2.14 Speech delay

1. A: Electroencephalogram (EEG)

The diagnosis of Landau–Kleffner syndrome should be considered in a child who loses language skills. The onset is usually between 3 and 9 years and is characterised by rapid loss of language skills after initial normal language development. There are typical EEG abnormalities, and the syndrome has a variable prognosis. Most patients will still have language difficulties as adults, ranging from those with almost no verbal ability to those with mild deficits in verbal communication.

2. C: Creatine kinase

This child is showing mild delay in all areas of his development, more marked in speech and language. The diagnosis that needs to be excluded is Duchenne muscular dystrophy, particularly as he only walked at 21 months. Boys with Duchenne muscular dystrophy usually have associated learning difficulties, and often present to the medical professional with concerns about speech and language before any muscle weakness is apparent.

3. G: Genetic studies for fragile X

This child is showing significant developmental delay in all areas of his development. He is also demonstrating some autistic features, with poor eye contact, chewing, and fiddling. The information about the uncle suggests a genetic disease such as fragile X. Duchenne muscular dystrophy is not likely, as affected individuals do not usually survive into their late 20s.

2.15 Children Act

1. G: Emergency Protection Order (EPO)

This order lasts for a maximum of 8 days, with a possibility of extension for a further 7 days. This order may be granted by the court if there is reason to believe that a child may be harmed if not removed from their present accommodation.

The Emergency Protection Order replaced the **Place of Safety Order**, and may be granted by the court if one of the following is satisfied:

- There is reasonable cause to believe that the child is likely to suffer appreciable harm if not removed from their present accommodation.
- Enquiries by the local authority are being frustrated by lack of access.

In addition, a child likely to suffer significant harm may also be taken into police protection for 72 hours using a **Police Protection Order**; this involves a decision internal to the police force, and is quicker than applying for an EPO.

2. B: Care Order

This order confers parental responsibility on the social services (in addition to that of the parents) and usually involves removal from home. It may be applied for in cases of non-accidental injury where enquires will take some time, and when the child is not regarded as being safe at home. Care orders can be taken out by a court if they are convinced that the threshold for appreciable harm to the child has been met.

3. D: Child Assessment Order

This order may be used if there is a situation of persistent but non-urgent suspicion of risk. It overrides the objections of a parent to whatever examination or assessment is needed to see whether the child is at significant harm. This order lasts up to 7 days.

A **Supervision Order** gives the social services the power and duty to visit the family and also to impose conditions, such as attendance at a clinic, nursery, school, or outpatient visits. If insufficient powers are available via the Children Act, then **Wardship** via the High Court may be applied for. This gives the court virtually unlimited powers, and is used in exceptional circumstances, such as when a family objects to medical treatment because of religious reasons. The **Statementing Order** does not exist.

3. Clinical Pharmacology and Toxicology

Multiple True–False Questions

3.1 Concerning the suitability of the excipients in a medicine for use in neonates,

- ☐ A benzyl alcohol should be avoided in injectable preparations
- ☐ B propylene glycol must be avoided at any concentration
- ☐ C lactose is contraindicated
- ☐ D sugar-free medicines are not essential
- ☐ E alcohol concentration can cause intoxication in infants

3.2 The following statements relating to paediatric dosing that requires alteration of a product designed for adults are true:

- ☐ A it is never acceptable to cut a coated tablet
- ☐ B dispersible tablets always form a uniform concentration when dissolved in water
- ☐ C injectable product may occasionally be administered orally
- ☐ D not all 'non-coated' tablets are dispersible in water
- ☐ E suppositories are easily cut to give accurate dosing to children

3.3 Concerning accurate paediatric dosing,

- ☐ A to obtain any child's dose, divide the adult dose by 70 and multiply by the child's weight
- ☐ B the surface area equates more accurately with the extracellular fluid than does weight
- ☐ C the adult dose is usually taken as the upper dose for children
- ☐ D doses should never be rounded to avoid using decimal points
- ☐ E adult dosing is always more logical than children's dosing

3.4 Prescribing outside a product licence:

- [ ] A it is poor practice to prescribe outside a licence
- [ ] B information from the manufacturer that must be given out with a product may state that the product is not suitable in children
- [ ] C all information in the *British National Formulary* (*BNF*) is covered by the licence
- [ ] D all information in the *BNF for Children* is covered by the licence
- [ ] E carers must give formal consent for children in their care to receive medicines that are outside their licence

3.5 Therapeutic drug monitoring may be indicated in the following circumstances:

- [ ] A to confirm toxicity
- [ ] B to check compliance
- [ ] C to confirm steady state
- [ ] D to monitor plasma levels if an interacting drug has been added
- [ ] E to monitor plasma levels of a hepatically cleared drug if renal function has changed

3.6 The following drug interactions are known:

- [ ] A phenytoin increases the plasma concentrations of theophylline
- [ ] B erythromycin increases the chances of bleeding in children stabilised on warfarin
- [ ] C carbamazepine is an enzyme inducer
- [ ] D girls taking the oral contraceptive pill may need extra protection if rifampicin is started
- [ ] E omeprazole can decrease the level of some drugs that are metabolised by the liver

Best of Five Questions

3.7   A neonate of 2 kg requires amphotericin B at a dose of 1 mg/kg
      to treat a systemic fungal infection. A single-lumen peripheral
      line is in situ. What would be the BEST option for administering
      the medicine?

☐   A   Insert a central line
☐   B   Mix the amphotericin with 0.9% sodium chloride
☐   C   Give the amphotericin undiluted
☐   D   Mix the amphotericin with 5% glucose
☐   E   Mix the amphotericin with 5% glucose and a buffer

3.8   A 5-year-old requires a dose of oral liquid nifedipine at a dose of
      5 mg twice a day. The preparations available to prescribe are:
      liquid-filled capsules, modified-release tablets, injection, and an
      imported liquid not licensed in the UK. What would be the BEST
      option for administering the nifedipine?

☐   A   Crush the tablets and sprinkle over food
☐   B   Crush the tablets and put in 5 mL of water
☐   C   Remove the liquid from the capsules
☐   D   Give the content of the injection orally
☐   E   Use the imported liquid which is not licensed in the UK

3.9   A pre-term neonate who weighs 2.5 kg and is 3 days old requires
      a higher dose of benzylpenicillin on a mg/kg basis than an adult
      to achieve the same plasma concentration. Which of the
      following BEST describes why this should be?

☐   A   Benzylpenicillin crosses the blood–brain barrier in neonates more
         readily
☐   B   Neonates have a greater volume of distribution for water-soluble
         drugs
☐   C   Benzylpenicillin is water-soluble and distributes to the kidneys at a
         faster rate in neonates
☐   D   Benzylpenicillin is excreted from the kidney more slowly in neonates
☐   E   The protein binding of benzylpenicillin is lower in neonates

3.10 The therapeutic plasma range of phenytoin is lower in neonates than in children. What is the MOST likely reason for this?

☐ A Less phenytoin is needed to treat seizures on a mg/kg basis
☐ B Bilirubin displaces phenytoin from albumin more readily in neonates
☐ C Decreased albumin levels lead to increased 'free' phenytoin
☐ D Phenytoin is more toxic in neonates
☐ E Phenytoin is excreted more slowly in neonates

3.11 Chloramphenicol may cause 'grey baby syndrome' in neonates. What is the MOST likely reason for this?

☐ A Chloramphenicol is able to cross the blood–brain barrier
☐ B Neonatal livers are unable to glucuronidate high doses of chloramphenicol
☐ C Chloramphenicol is glucuronidated to a toxic metabolite in neonates
☐ D Grey baby syndrome is an idiosyncratic reaction to chloramphenicol in neonates
☐ E At birth, neonatal sulfation is more established than is glucuronidation

3.12 A neonate born at 37 weeks of gestation presents at 2 weeks old. The baby was commenced on phenytoin 2 days previously and the plasma level of phenytoin 8 hours post-dose was 8 mg/L. At presentation the infant is still having seizures. What would be the MOST appropriate clinical approach?

☐ A Leave the prescription the same, because steady state hasn't been reached
☐ B Double the dose and monitor in another 3 days
☐ C Increase the dose by about 20% and monitor the child
☐ D Monitor the albumin to see if it is a true level
☐ E Stop the phenytoin and start another anticonvulsant

3.13 A 10-kg 14-month-old boy is brought to the accident and emergency department by his parents. His parents claim that he possibly ingested paracetamol, as six 500-mg capsules were found to be missing from the family's paracetamol container. This possible ingestion occurred within a 60-minute window before their presentation to the Emergency Department. Of the five choices below, which is the MOST appropriate immediate management action?

- ☐ A Measure plasma paracetamol levels
- ☐ B Administer ipecacuanha to induce emesis
- ☐ C Perform a gastric lavage
- ☐ D Administer *N*-acetylcysteine
- ☐ E Administer activated charcoal

Extended Matching Questions

3.14 Theme: Interactions

A Drug / drug
B Drug / diluent
C Drug / flush
D Drug / plastic
E Drug / acid
F Drug / food
G Drug / water
H Drug / alkali

For each of the scenarios below, select the most likely interaction to account for the loss of efficacy of the drug. Each option may be used once, more than once, or not at all.

- ☐ 1. Gentamicin is being given to a neonate for a Gram-negative infection. After the addition of benzylpenicillin co-administered down the same line, the levels of gentamicin are decreased.
- ☐ 2. A child receives insulin that was mixed in a 500-mL bag of sodium chloride. Over the course of 24 hours, the insulin becomes less effective.
- ☐ 3. A child is receiving omeprazole tablets that are crushed and dissolved in water before administration. A nasogastric tube becomes necessary during the child's management. After its insertion, the effect of the administered omeprazole is seen to be much less than before the tube was inserted.

3.15 Theme: Neonatal pharmacology

A   Gut motility
B   Gut acidity
C   Hepatic glucuronidation
D   Hepatic sulfation
E   Renal function
F   Protein binding
G   Volume of distribution
H   Permeability of the blood–brain barrier

Select the process which is most likely to be altered (from that of children and adults) and so be responsible for the following situations in neonates. Each option may be used once, more than once, or not at all.

☐ 1. A 2-week-old term baby requires a higher dose (on a mg/kg basis) of a water-soluble drug in order to achieve the same plasma concentration.

☐ 2. Addition of co-trimoxazole to a neonate with high plasma levels of bilirubin can quickly become life-threatening.

☐ 3. Dosing of benzylpenicillin in a 1-week-old, 30-week gestation neonate is usually at a frequency of two or three times a day, as opposed to four times a day in children.

MT–F Answers

3.1 Drug excipients: A E

Benzyl alcohol can cause severe respiratory problems in neonates, and thus should be avoided. Some medicines contain so much alcohol that even normal doses in the very young can cause intoxication. Propylene glycol is hypertonic, and fast administration of high quantities can cause haemodynamic instability. However, small amounts infused slowly are acceptable. Lactose may be used in any patient, providing they are not lactose intolerant. Sugar-free medicines are desirable in all children, because sugar can cause dental caries; however, the administration of small amounts of sugar-containing medicines for short periods of time is acceptable.

3.2 Alteration of a product for paediatric dosing: C D

Although it is rarely desirable, injectable products may occasionally be used orally or intranasally, although the pH often means that the liquid is not very palatable. Plain tablets with no special release mechanisms may be suitable for crushing, but the particles may not disperse in water at all, leaving all the particles on the bottom of the vessel. It is never desirable to cut a coated tablet, but in the absence of any other product it may be acceptable, if the coat has no modifying-release properties such as a basic sugar coat. Just because a tablet is dispersible, it doesn't mean that it dissolves to form a uniform solution. Suppositories may not have the medication dispersed evenly throughout the product, and thus cutting is not desirable in terms of accurate dosing.

3.3 Paediatric dosing: B C

Most drugs are distributed in the extracellular fluid, and so basing dosing on a child:adult surface area ratio of an adult dose is more accurate than using a weight ratio, as the extracellular fluid is more closely related to the surface area than to the weight. Although some children may theoretically require larger doses than an adult because of their size and liver function, the adult dose is usually taken as the maximum dose. Most adults get the same dose of a drug independent of their size (eg paracetamol); their plasma levels may therefore vary enormously. Dosing like this only works because most drugs have wide therapeutic ranges. Because of the wide therapeutic ranges, rounding of doses to avoid decimal points is usually good practice; however, this sometimes causes large variance in doses, and might not be acceptable for dosing within a narrow therapeutic range.

3.4   Prescribing outside a product licence: B

Prescribers can prescribe irrespective of whether something has a licence or not, but the prescriber must be aware of the clinical evidence and the quality of the product they are prescribing. A company's patient information leaflets must legally be given out with a licensed product, even if it is contrary to what the product is being used for. Most information in the *BNF* is covered by the manufacturer's licence, but not all. The *BNF for Children* contains a lot more information that is not covered by the licence. It is good practice to discuss with a patient all their medicines and their evidence base.

3.5   Therapeutic drug monitoring: A B D

Therapeutic drug monitoring should only be carried out if there is a real need to do so. Toxicity is often diagnosed by symptoms, and can occur at normal plasma levels. However, if toxicity is expected, therapeutic drug monitoring should be carried out to ascertain the current level. If non-compliance is expected, therapeutic drug monitoring may confirm the situation. If a patient is stable and their plasma levels known, then therapeutic drug monitoring should be carried out after an interacting medicine has been added, to observe what is happening to the patient. Steady state is a stable plasma level reached after about 5 half-lives of the drug. Therapeutic drug monitoring is normally carried out after steady state has been reached, rather than to confirm steady state. If a drug is hepatically cleared, its levels should not be altered if renal function changes, and thus no additional monitoring is needed.

3.6   Drug interactions: B C D

Erythromycin is an enzyme inhibitor and thus increases the levels of warfarin, leading to potential bleeding. Carbamazepine is an enzyme inducer. Rifampicin is an enzyme inducer that increases the metabolism of the oral contraceptive pill, leading to a greater chance of conception. Phenytoin is an enzyme inducer, and thus decreases the levels of the hepatically cleared theophylline. Omeprazole is a weak enzyme inhibitor, and thus increases the levels of some drugs that are metabolised by the liver.

Best of Five Answers

3.7   E: Mix the amphotericin with 5% glucose and a buffer

Amphotericin B does not need to be administered through a central line, although if treatment is long-term it may be preferable. It must be diluted and given as an infusion. It is not stable in acid solutions, so 5% glucose is not appropriate; however, it reacts with chloride ions, making it incompatible with sodium chloride. Ideally, it is put in glucose that has been neutralised with buffer, and this is the normal method of administration.

3.8   E: Use the imported liquid which is not licensed in the UK

Sprinkling crushed tablets over food for children is not advisable, as not all the food may be eaten. Crushing the modified-release tablets in water will change the properties of the modified release, but also these tablets don't disperse very well, and thus the whole dose may not be given. The liquid may be withdrawn from the capsules, but this is a difficult process and knowledge is needed of how much of the liquid holds the actual dose, and this will vary with different brands. It may be possible to give the injection orally, but this is expensive and not at all pleasant. An imported product that is licensed in its country of origin is often the best option, providing care is taken if documents need translation.

3.9   B: Neonates have a greater volume of distribution for water-soluble drugs

All the answers are true for benzylpenicillin in the neonate, but the reason for the higher dose is only due to the higher volume of distribution caused by the increased extracellular fluid.

3.10 C: Decreased albumin levels lead to increased 'free' phenytoin

The main reason for the lower plasma phenytoin levels is the decreased albumin concentrations. The phenytoin excretion is reasonable from birth. Albumin binding is not as tight as it is in children, but bilirubin rarely plays a part in displacing large amounts, unless levels are very high. The overall plasma concentration of phenytoin needs to be lower because there is more free (non-bound) drug and thus dosing can be reduced compared with that in adults and children.

3.11 B: Neonatal livers are unable to glucuronidate high doses of chloramphenicol

Glucuronidation is one of the last metabolic processes to be established in neonates. Some drugs are sulfated in preference, but chloramphenicol is not. Thus high doses of chloramphenicol are not able to be metabolised, and toxic levels pass into the central nervous system and other organs, to produce the often fatal effects of the grey baby syndrome.

3.12 C: Increase the dose by about 20% and monitor the child

Phenytoin demonstrates saturable kinetics within the therapeutic range (10–20 mg/L). This means that large dose adjustments just outside the range or within the range are likely to lead to very large variations in plasma levels and to render the child toxic. Although the levels are likely to increase a little over the next few days until steady state is reached, this is unlikely to be adequate or fast enough for this patient. Albumin may well be affecting the level, but the patient needs to be treated now, irrespective of the amount of free phenytoin. Doubling or re-loading the patient should only be considered in an emergency.

3.13 E: Administer activated charcoal

The most appropriate management in this instance would be to administer activated charcoal, to limit further absorption of paracetamol. Inducing emesis with ipecacuanha is now generally contraindicated. Measurement of plasma paracetamol levels is useful only after 4 hours of ingestion. A gastric lavage may be beneficial, but when you are given these five choices it would not be the first choice of treatment. N-Acetylcysteine would not be the first line of treatment either.

EMQ Answers

3.14 Interactions

1. A: Drug / drug

Penicillins interact with gentamicin if they come into contact, and the gentamicin is degraded.

2. D: Drug / plastic

Insulin is absorbed onto plastic and, over time, the amount in the bag is decreased. For this reason, insulin is usually given via a syringe driver.

3. E: Drug / acid

Omeprazole tablets are made of tiny spheres of coated drug. The drug is absorbed in the duodenum but is degraded by acid. The spheres' coats are thus acid-resistant. If they are crushed, the drug will be degraded by the stomach acid, making it less effective. The crushed tablets are sometimes given mixed with sodium bicarbonate to try to protect the drug.

3.15 Neonatal pharmacology

1. G: Volume of distribution

Neonates have a far greater relative extracellular fluid volume than infants (who have a far greater relative fat content), so neonates require relatively more water-soluble drug to achieve the same plasma concentration.

2. H: Permeability of the blood–brain barrier

Co-trimoxazole can displace bilirubin from its albumin-binding sites in any individual. However, this event can quickly become life-threatening in a neonate. The blood–brain barrier is very permeable, and allows the increased bilirubin across into the brain. If this happens, the often fatal encephalopathy of kernicterus will occur.

3. E: Renal function

Benzylpenicillin is cleared renally. Neonates have a reduced renal clearance and they do not require such frequent dosing, despite requiring the same doses (if not higher) on a mg/kg basis.

4. Dermatology

Multiple True–False Questions

4.1   The normal procedure for a skin biopsy involves

☐ A   oral sedation
☐ B   uninvolved skin
☐ C   taking an elliptical piece of skin and suturing the wound
☐ D   a special technique for epidermolysis bullosa
☐ E   a scar being left in 50% of cases

4.2   The following are true of skin infections:

☐ A   they are usually caused by *Staphylococcus epidermidis*
☐ B   nodules may persist for 3 months after successful treatment of scabies
☐ C   tinea infections are usually due to *Microsporum canis*
☐ D   tinea corporis will show improvement if steroid creams are applied
☐ F   scalp abscesses due to fungal infection require incision and drainage

4.3   The following conditions are more common in children with atopic eczema:

☐ A   juvenile plantar dermatosis
☐ B   lamellar ichthyosis
☐ C   cataracts
☐ D   pityriasis alba
☐ E   keratosis pilaris

4.4   In infected atopic eczema, the following is true:

☐ A   steroid creams/ointments should be stopped in eczema herpeticum
☐ B   wet wraps are an effective treatment for infected eczema
☐ C   eczema herpeticum is treated with intravenous aciclovir
☐ D   failure to respond to a course of oral antibiotics is the result of methicillin-resistant *Staphylococcus aureus* (MRSA) infection
☐ E   topical antibiotic is the treatment of choice

4.5   Blisters are found in the following conditions:

☐ A   toxic epidermal necrolysis
☐ B   erythema multiforme
☐ C   erythropoietic protoporphyria
☐ D   Stevens–Johnson syndrome
☐ E   granuloma annulare

4.6   Nail changes are a recognised feature of:

☐ A   epidermolysis bullosa
☐ B   hypothyroidism
☐ C   pityriasis rubra pilaris
☐ D   alopecia areata
☐ E   atopic eczema

Best of Five Questions

4.7   A 2-year-old boy presents to the casualty department with a 3-day history of a high temperature and widespread erythematous skin, with peeling skin on the fingers. Which of the following treatments is MOST appropriate?

☐ A   Morphine
☐ B   Flucloxacillin
☐ C   Aciclovir
☐ D   Methotrexate
☐ E   Immunoglobulins

4.8   Since she was 6 months of age, a 2-year-old girl has been affected by an itchy red rash of the limb flexures, which comes and goes. Which would be the MOST suitable initial treatment?

☐ A   Diet free from cow's milk
☐ B   Betnovate cream applied twice daily
☐ C   Use of regular emollient therapy
☐ D   Pimecrolimus cream (1%) applied to the face
☐ E   Tacrolimus ointment (0.03%)

4.9 An 8-year-old girl has severe generalised atopic eczema and has attended clinic monthly for the last 6 months. She has missed nearly 4 weeks of school in the past 2 months. Which treatment would be MOST appropriate?

- [ ] A   Twice-daily application of emollient wet wraps
- [ ] B   Twice-daily application of clobetasone (Eumovate) cream
- [ ] C   Oral acitretin
- [ ] D   Oral ciclosporin
- [ ] E   Twice-daily application of clobetasol (Dermovate) cream

4.10 A 9-year-old girl has had widespread plaque psoriasis for the past 3 years, affecting her limbs, trunk, and face. Many treatments have been tried without success. She has missed several weeks of school and has regularly attended the dermatology clinic. Which of the following therapies is the MOST appropriate?

- [ ] A   Psoralen ultraviolet A (PUVA)
- [ ] B   Vitamin D analogues
- [ ] C   Betnovate 1 in 4 cream
- [ ] D   Methotrexate
- [ ] E   Penicillin V

4.11 A 6-year-old girl complains of a red scaly rash on the limbs. On examination, you find numerous plaques affecting the arms and legs. Which of the following is MOST likely?

- [ ] A   Onset of rash was in the first 2 years of life
- [ ] B   Rubbing the skin provokes white scaling
- [ ] C   Oral lesions with a white reticulate surface
- [ ] D   Flexural sites are affected
- [ ] E   Severe destructive arthritis that symmetrically affects large joints

4.12 An 18-month-old boy is referred by his GP with a 5-day history of not eating and drinking, being unwell, and having multiple mouth and lip ulcers, and white lesions on the tongue. This is his first attendance at the surgery because of illness. On examination, he has a pulse rate of 120 beats/min, a blood pressure of 85/55 mmHg, and his capillary refill time is less than 2 seconds. Which of the following is MOST important for his care?

- [ ] A   Oral nystatin
- [ ] B   Regular mouth care, including antiseptic mouthwashes
- [ ] C   Intravenous aciclovir
- [ ] D   Intravenous fluids
- [ ] E   Oral paracetamol

4.13 A 13-month-old boy has an itchy red rash and coryzal symptoms. Which one of the following is MOST likely?

☐ A   The pattern of rash is helpful in making the diagnosis
☐ B   The rash will have resolved within a week
☐ C   An urticarial rash rarely occurs with viral infections
☐ D   The season may give a clue to the diagnosis
☐ E   A causal agent is identified in 75% of cases

Extended Matching Questions

4.14 Theme: Skin rashes and viral infections

A   Rubella
B   Scarlet fever
C   Non-specific viral exanthema
D   Roseola infantum
E   Erythema infectiosum
F   Gianotti–Crosti syndrome
G   Herpes simplex virus
H   Coxsackie infection

For each child described below with a viral infection and skin lesions, select the most likely condition from the list above. Each option may be used once, more than once, or not at all.

☐ 1. An 18-month-old girl presents with a 2-week history of erythematous papules that started on the upper legs and buttocks, and then spread to the arms and cheeks.
☐ 2. A 2-year-old girl presents with a 3-day history of a high temperature and malaise, with vesicles in the mouth and on her thumb.
☐ 3. A 9-month-old boy presents with a convulsion. He has had a high temperature for 4 days, suboccipital lymph nodes, and has a pink macular rash that started on the trunk and spread to the extremities.

4.15 Theme: Vesiculopustular lesions

A Impetigo
B Transient neonatal pustulosis
C Scabies
D Erythema toxicum neonatorum
E Urticaria pigmentosa
F Epidermolysis bullosa
G Infantile acropustulosis
H Incontinentia pigmenti

For each infant described below with a vesiculopustular rash, select the condition that is most likely from the above list. Each option may be used once, more than once, or not at all.

☐ 1. A 1-week-old girl is noticed to have vesicular lesions which spare her face. Examination shows that she is apyrexial, and the lesions follow Blaschko's lines and are in a linear distribution on the limbs and arranged circumferentially on the trunk.

☐ 2. An 8-month-old girl presents with a 6-month history of crops of itchy small vesicopustules on the hands and feet recurring at monthly intervals.

☐ 3. A West Indian baby girl is noticed to have vesicopustules at birth, some of which have burst, leaving a pigmented macule.

MT–F Answers

4.1 Skin biopsy: D

In epidermolysis bullosa, a shave biopsy is taken after rubbing unaffected skin. For a skin biopsy, a 3- or 4-mm punch biopsy carried out under local anaesthesia is the normal procedure. Elliptical pieces of skin are taken often as part of cot death investigations and when an excision biopsy is needed. Usually, affected skin is chosen, but unaffected skin is required for some conditions, eg direct immunofluorescence in linear IgA disease (chronic bullous dermatosis of childhood) and for epidermolysis bullosa. Although a scar may be left by a punch biopsy (eg in a child who has previously had hypertrophic scars or keloids), in the majority of cases the biopsy site heals well, leaving no long-term scar.

4.2 Skin infections: B D

Skin infections in an immunocompetent child are usually caused by *Staphylococcus aureus* or group A β-haemolytic *Streptococcus*. Scabetic nodules are the result of an immune response to the mite, and often persist for 2–3 months after successful treatment. If new lesions appear, then treatment has not been successful. The majority of tinea infections are due to *Trichophyton* species, with human-to-human spread, rather than *Microsporum* from animals. Tinea corporis does show temporary improvement with topical steroid creams, as the redness and inflammation improve. Pustules are often prominent and the edge of the lesion is less scaly. The appearance is given the term 'tinea incognito'. Scalp abscesses due to fungal infection are called kerions. These should not be incised and drained, as a permanent scar will be left. The treatment of choice is antifungal therapy started without delay.

4.3 Conditions associated with atopic eczema: A C D E

All the conditions except for lamellar ichthyosis are more common in children with atopic eczema. Atopic eczema is, however, associated with ichthyosis vulgaris, which is the most common form of ichthyosis, with an incidence of 1 in 250; it is characterised by fine, light, scaly skin, in contrast to the large, dark plate-like scales of lamellar ichthyosis. Juvenile plantar dermatosis affects the sole of the foot, with red, shiny skin, often with painful fissures. Anterior subcapsular cataracts affect 4–12% of children with atopic eczema. Posterior subcapsular cataracts are due to use of either oral corticosteroids or topical steroid creams or ointments applied to the eyelids or around the eye. In pityriasis alba there are dry, slightly scaly hypopigmented areas, common on the face and upper trunk. Keratosis pilaris is keratin plugging of hair follicles, with varying degrees of surrounding erythema that tends to be prominent on the upper arms and legs.

4.4 Infected atopic eczema: A C

Steroid creams or ointments should be discontinued in eczema herpeticum, as they are thought to encourage viral spread. Most cases are due to widespread infection of the skin with herpes simplex virus, and need intravenous aciclovir. Wet wraps should be discontinued if there is overt skin infection. There are many reasons why children do not respond to a course of oral antibiotics, eg too short a course given (10 days is treatment duration of choice), flucloxacillin only given, and group A β-haemolytic *Streptococcus* is present in addition to *Staphylococcus aureus*, erythromycin resistance, nasal *Staphylococcus* carriage. MRSA colonisation of eczema is increasing amongst children with chronic eczema – remember that whether to treat is a clinical decision, as most children with atopic eczema have positive skin swabs for *S. aureus*. Infection is usually widespread, and needs oral antibiotics rather than topical ones. Use of topical antibiotics is for localised infections only, and those such as fusidic acid (Fucidin) should not be used for more than 5 days; otherwise bacterial resistance occurs.

4.5 Conditions associated with blisters: A B D

In both toxic epidermal necrolysis and Stevens–Johnson syndrome, there is erythematous skin with bullae. Erythema multiforme characteristically has symmetrical red papules with target lesions, some of which may blister. In erythropoeitic protoporphyria there is photosensitivity and small pitted scars on the cheeks, which should not be confused with eczema; blistering is not a typical feature. In granuloma annulare, lesions are ring-shaped, with skin-coloured papules but not blisters.

4.6 Nail changes: All true

Epidermolysis bullosa is the name given to a group of genetically determined disorders in which the skin and mucosae are excessively susceptible to separation from the underlying tissues and blistering following trauma. Nails may be affected in both junctional and dystrophic epidermolysis bullosa. In hypothyroidism there is decreased nail growth, ridging and brittleness. Pityriasis rubra pilaris is an erythematous eruption of unknown aetiology characterised by palmoplantar keratoderma (thickening of skin on palms and soles). There are different types, with nail features that include thickened curved nails and terminal hyperaemia (half-and-half nail). Nail changes in alopecia areata are usually in the form of nail pitting. Such changes tend to be greater in those with more severe disease. In atopic eczema there may be nail pitting, Beau's lines, and onycholysis (separation of the nail plate from the nail bed).

Best of Five Answers

4.7   B: Flucloxacillin

This is staphylococcal scalded-skin syndrome. Systemic antibiotics are needed. Although uncomfortable, pain relief with paracetamol / ibuprofen is usually sufficient. Morphine is required in Stevens–Johnson syndrome or toxic epidermal necrolysis. Aciclovir would be given for herpes simplex virus (HSV) infection when lesions at different stages would be expected in addition to erythema. Peeling is not usually found in HSV infection. Methotrexate would be indicated for acute erythrodermic psoriasis. Infection must always be excluded before making this diagnosis, and a skin biopsy is recommended. Immunoglobulins would be given for Kawasaki disease; for this diagnosis, 5 days of fever is required, and skin peeling is a late sign, typically in the second week.

4.8   C: Use of regular emollient therapy

This is atopic eczema. It is the initial treatment that is being considered, and this should include use of emollients such as bath oils, soap substitutes and moisturisers. A diet free of cow's milk may be considered for severe atopic eczema, especially in those younger than 1 year of age. Betamethasone (Betnovate) cream is a potent topical steroid that is not used routinely in the treatment of childhood atopic eczema. Both topical pimecrolimus and tacrolimus are used for treatment of moderate to severe eczema that is not responding to conventional treatment.

4.9   D: Oral ciclosporin

This is chronic atopic eczema that is evidently not responding to treatment, as the girl is coming to clinic monthly and is taking a lot of time off school. A short course of oral ciclosporin is one of the systemic therapies used for atopic eczema not responding to topical therapies. Emollient wet wraps may help as part of the treatment regimen, but other therapy is needed, and wet wraps are often not well tolerated by older children. Clobetasone (Eumovate) cream is a moderately potent topical steroid cream which would already have been used in this case. Acitretin is used in the treatment of psoriasis and ichthyotic disorders. Clobetasol (Dermovate) cream is a potent topical steroid cream. Potent steroid creams should be used cautiously in children because of possible local skin side-effects and, as the eczema is generalised, there should be concern about the child developing Cushing syndrome.

4.10 D: Methotrexate

This is chronic plaque psoriasis which is relapsing often, and which is not under control. Many topical therapies will have been used over a 3-year period. Systemic therapy is warranted, and methotrexate is one of the systemic drugs used for psoriasis. PUVA involves the use of phytotoxic psoralens in combination with ultraviolet A light, and tends not to be used in children (particularly in those younger than teenagers) because its use increases the risk of skin cancer. Vitamin D analogues (eg calcipotriol [Dovonex]) are used for mild to moderate psoriasis when less than 40% of the skin area is affected. Penicillin V is used in the treatment of guttate psoriasis, which may be triggered by streptococcal infection, and in other forms of psoriasis only if there is evidence of streptococcal infection.

4.11 B: Rubbing the skin provokes white scaling

This is chronic plaque psoriasis. If erythematous plaques are present and are due to psoriasis, then rubbing produces the typical white scale. Less than 2% of psoriasis presents in the first 2 years of life and 10% of cases will have an age of onset less than 10 years. Girls tend to be affected between the ages of 5 and 9 years and boys between 15 and 19 years. Lesions in the mouth affecting the buccal mucosa with a white reticulate surface are typical of lichen planus. Psoriasis tends to affect the extensor surfaces. Psoriatic arthritis is occasionally severely destructive. It tends to be an asymmetric arthritis.

4.12 E: Oral paracetamol

This is primary herpes simplex gingivostomatitis. Pain relief is needed, and paracetamol is appropriate. The tongue is often white, and this is not usually due to *Candida*. Mouth care is difficult to perform in children, and most mouthwashes sting, causing further misery to the child. Aciclovir stops further viral replication, but does not help when there are several lesions present. Some children treated with aciclovir develop poorer antibody responses. This child is highly unlikely to be immunocompromised or to have skin disease, as it is his first attendance at the GP surgery. Intravenous fluids may be needed in very severe cases, but children often start to drink after adequate analgesia has been given.

4.13 D: The season may give a clue to the diagnosis

Some infections are more common in certain seasons, eg enteroviruses are more common in summer and autumn. The pattern of rash may be helpful in making a diagnosis (as in hand, foot and mouth disease), but is often non-specific in the majority of cases of viral rash. Rashes associated with viral infections can last for 2–3 weeks, and sometimes longer. Urticarial rashes occur quite often with viral infections. Most viral rashes are not investigated, and would tend to be only if atypical or if the child had been in contact with a pregnant mother or immunocompromised child or adult.

EMQ Answers

4.14 Skin rashes and viral infections

1.   F: Gianotti–Crosti syndrome

Gianotti–Crosti syndrome (also known as papular acrodermatitis) typically occurs in children of 1–6 years of age. Symmetrical lichenoid, skin-coloured or coppery-red papules develop and last 3–6 weeks. Lesions are on the legs and buttocks, and then spread to the arms and face. It is important to recognise this condition because of the duration of the rash. Many viruses have been linked to Gianotti–Crosti syndrome. In scarlet fever, the rash starts in the axillae and groins and consists of fine, red papules. The erythroderma fades over 2–3 days, followed by desquamation 7–10 days later.

2.   G: Herpes simplex virus

In primary HSV infection, children are febrile, miserable, and may have several mouth lesions. HSV lesions on the digits are common, because children suck their fingers (and toes). In hand, foot and mouth disease caused by coxsackie infection, the fever is low-grade.

3.   D: Roseola infantum

Children with roseola infantum (synonyms – exanthema subitum, sixth disease) are typically aged between 6 and 36 months and have 3–5 days of high fever, with enlarged suboccipital lymph nodes. The rose-pink rash tends to last for 2 days, starting on the trunk and then spreading to the extremities and the face. Once the rash comes out, the temperature becomes normal. Human herpesvirus types 6 and 7 have been found in this condition. In rubella there is lymphadenopathy – especially cervical, postauricular and suboccipital – but fever is low-grade and it is not associated with convulsions. Fever occurs for 1–2 days in erythema infectiosum (slapped-cheek disease) caused by parvovirus infection and there is a generalised maculopapular exanthem, which is often 'lace-like', on the limbs after physical activity.

4.15 Vesiculopustular lesions

1. H: Incontinentia pigmenti

Incontinentia pigmenti is an X-linked dominant condition and is usually lethal in boys. Lesions typically develop in the first week of life, and the first stage is a vesicular one. Had widespread impetigo been present, the baby would be expected to have systemic symptoms, including pyrexia. It is rather early for a scabies rash to develop, and this rash does not follow Blaschko's lines. Lesions are papules as well as vesicles. Erythema toxicum neonatorum does not follow Blaschko's lines. Epidermolysis bullosa often presents at birth with absence of skin.

2. G: Infantile acropustulosis

Infantile acropustulosis usually presents in the first few months of life and is characterised by recurrent crops of vesicopustules on the hands and feet.

3. B: Transient neonatal pustulosis

Transient neonatal pustulosis is characterised by pustules present at birth, some of which may have ruptured. They leave a pigmented macule, which may persist for up to 3 months. It is more common in black skin. Urticaria pigmentosa commonly presents in the first year of life but can be present at birth. These are skin-coloured or red–brown macules which urticate when rubbed.

5. Emergency Medicine

Multiple True–False Questions

5.1   The basic life support algorithm includes the following:

☐ A   two rescue breaths are administered before chest compressions are commenced

☐ B   agonal breaths may be present in the child with cardiac arrest

☐ C   the femoral pulse is recommended to check for circulation in children

☐ D   compressions should be at a rate of 80 per minute

☐ E   emergency services should be called after 1 minute of cardiopulmonary resuscitation (CPR)

5.2   In the case of asystole,

☐ A   the initial dose of adrenaline is 0.1 mL/kg of 1 in 1000 adrenaline

☐ B   repeat doses of adrenaline are 0.1 mL/kg of 1 in 1000 adrenaline

☐ C   in a neonate, adrenaline should be given down the endotracheal tube

☐ D   in hospital, the ratio of compressions to ventilation for a 7-year-old is 30:2

☐ E   as soon as the child's trachea is intubated, continuous chest compressions can be commenced

5.3   Pulseless electrical activity

☐ A   is a shockable rhythm

☐ B   has a rhythm on the monitor that is indistinguishable from ventricular tachycardia

☐ C   is a rhythm that may be seen in a patient with hypovolaemia

☐ D   requires that a shock of 4 J/kg be given

☐ E   may be seen in a child with a pulmonary embolus

5.4   The following is true in cases of choking:

☐ A   for the choking child, chest thrusts should be used instead of abdominal thrusts

☐ B   back blows and chest thrusts should be at a rate of 1 per second

☐ C   a blind finger sweep may be performed before back blows

☐ D   the Heimlich procedure may be useful in an infant

☐ E   an effective cough should be encouraged

5.5   Which of the following statements is true of hypothermia?

☐ A   below 30°C, repeated shocks may be needed to treat ventricular fibrillation

☐ B   clotting is typically deranged in hypothermia

☐ C   during rewarming, fluid resuscitation should be avoided

☐ D   analgesia is recommended when rewarming is done in the presence of frostbite

☐ E   myocardial dysfunction may only become apparent on rewarming

5.6   With respect to electrocution injury,

☐ A   electrocution occurring outside the home is usually associated with other injuries

☐ B   dysrhythmias are a recognised late complication

☐ C   fluid and blood have the most resistance to electricity

☐ D   compartment syndrome is a recognised complication

☐ E   lightning injury is difficult to diagnose if not witnessed

5.7   When brainstem testing is performed,

☐ A   the recorded time of death follows the second set of tests

☐ B   the procedure is contraindicated to determine brainstem death in premature neonates

☐ C   two doctors with at least 5 years of post-qualification experience are required

☐ D   oculovestibular reflexes are no longer included

☐ E   death is pronounced after the second set of tests

Best of Five Questions

5.8   Which one of the following is the MOST correct concerning myoglobinuria?

☐ A   It is a rare complication of hypoxia

☐ B   Diuretics are relatively contraindicated

☐ C   Keeping the urine acid keeps the toxin in its ionised form

☐ D   Alkalinising the urine reduces the amount of resorption in the renal tubule

☐ E   The use of sodium bicarbonate should be avoided

5.9 Which one of the following statements is correct regarding airway resistance?

- [ ] A It is directly proportional to the radius squared
- [ ] B It is directly proportional to the radius to the power of 4
- [ ] C It is inversely proportional to the radius to the power of 4
- [ ] D It is inversely proportional to the radius squared
- [ ] E It is inversely proportional to the radius

5.10 In burns, which one of the following indications does not merit referral to a burns unit in a child?

- [ ] A An 8% partial-thickness burn to leg
- [ ] B A 6% full-thickness burn to arm
- [ ] C A 3% full-thickness burn to hands
- [ ] D A high-voltage burn to arm
- [ ] E A circumferential burn of one arm

5.11 Which one of the following interventions is not a recognised neuroprotective treatment following head injury?

- [ ] A Draining cerebrospinal fluid from a ventricular drain
- [ ] B Raising the head 20–30 degrees and keeping it in the midline
- [ ] C Aiming for high serum sodium levels (greater than 140 mmol/L)
- [ ] D Hyperventilation aiming for a PCO_2 between 3 and 3.5 kPa
- [ ] E Tight control of glucose using insulin for high glucose levels

5.12 Which one of the following statements is correct concerning inhaled nitric oxide?

- [ ] A It relaxes vascular and smooth muscle by stimulating production of cyclic adenosine monophosphate (cAMP)
- [ ] B It has marked effects on both pulmonary and peripheral vasculature
- [ ] C It suppresses endogenous release of nitric oxide from the respiratory mucosa
- [ ] D It rarely improves oxygenation in neonates with severe neonatal pulmonary hypertension
- [ ] E It rarely induces tolerance to its effects

5.13 With regard to the epidemiology of sepsis in children, which one of the following statements is correct?

- [ ] A Adolescents have the highest incidence of sepsis
- [ ] B The hospital mortality rate for children with severe sepsis is 30%
- [ ] C The mortality of severe sepsis in adults is three times that in children
- [ ] D Pre-existing morbidity is rare in those presenting with sepsis
- [ ] E Cardiac failure is a rare cause of death in those with severe sepsis

Extended Matching Questions

5.14 Theme: Airway obstruction

A Croup
B Epiglottitis
C Diphtheria
D Anaphylaxis
E Mediastinal tumour
F Inhaled foreign body
G Bacterial tracheitis
H Angioneurotic oedema
I Retropharyngeal abscess
J Asthma
K Tracheobronchomalacia

For each of the case histories below, select from the above causes of airways obstruction the one that best matches the clinical scenario. Each option may be used once, more than once, or not at all.

☐ 1. A 3-year-old child presents to the emergency department with a sudden onset of stridor, and a pyrexia of 40 °C. He is quiet and withdrawn. The mother informs you that her son has not been vaccinated.

☐ 2. A 15-year-old boy presents with difficulty breathing and a severe wheeze. A chest X-ray demonstrates hyperinflation and a widened mediastinum.

☐ 3. A 2-month-old girl with tetralogy of Fallot is noted to have a prolonged expiratory phase and is breathless. She has marked recession when she starts to cry. Her recession improves after nasal continuous positive airways pressure is commenced.

5.15 Theme: Adrenaline (epinephrine)

A   1 mg of intravenous adrenaline before the fourth shock
B   0.01 mL/kg of 1 in 10 000 adrenaline intravenously
C   5 mL of 1 in 1000 adrenaline via a nebuliser
D   1 mL of 1 in 1000 adrenaline via a nebuliser
E   0.1 mL/kg of 1 in 10 000 adrenaline via a nebuliser
F   0.1 mL/kg of 1 in 1000 adrenaline intramuscularly
G   0.01 mL/kg of 1 in 1000 adrenaline intramuscularly
H   0.1 mL/kg of 1 in 10 000 adrenaline intravenously before the third shock
I   0.1 mL/kg of 1 in 10 000 adrenaline intravenously before the second shock
J   infusion of adrenaline 1 µg/kg per min intravenously
K   0.05 mL/kg of 1 in 10 000 adrenaline intravenously
L   0.3 mL of 1 in 1000 adrenaline intramuscularly

For each of the following clinical scenarios, select from the above the most appropriate therapy. Each option may be used once, more than once, or not at all.

☐   1. A 3-year-old girl presents to the emergency department with severe croup. You are waiting for a senior anaesthetist to arrive, and they have suggested giving the child some adrenaline.

☐   2. An 8-year-old boy with a known nut allergy has been at a friend's party and eaten some chocolate cake. He has acute wheeze, is warm peripherally, and is tachycardic and hypotensive.

☐   3. A 10-year-old boy presents in the emergency department in ventricular fibrillation.

MT–F Answers

5.1 The basic life support algorithm: B E

A child, like an adult, may still have gasping respirations or agonal gasps during cardiac arrest, so the new algorithm asks lay people to check whether the child is breathing normally. The resuscitation team should be called after 1 minute of CPR. A rescue breath is a mouth to mouth and nose ventilation, or bag and mask assisted breaths given to a child who is not breathing. Five rescue breaths remain in the paediatric algorithm, because hypoxia is still the most common cause of paediatric arrest. The new guidelines suggest five rescue breaths as opposed to the previous advice of two effective breaths or five attempts at rescue breaths. The basic life support algorithm places more emphasis on looking for signs of circulation such as movement, coughing or normal breathing. Healthcare professionals who are trained and experienced are advised to check the brachial pulse in an infant and the carotid pulse in a child. Compressions should be at the rate of 100 per minute.

5.2 Asystole: E

As soon as intubation with an endotracheal tube has been achieved, continuous compressions can be commenced. In cardiac arrest, all doses of adrenaline are 0.1 mL/kg of 1 in 10 000 adrenaline. The endotracheal route is now not recommended for adrenaline in the newborn. The ratio of compressions to ventilations in hospital is 15:2. Out of hospital, those who are not healthcare professionals are recommended to use the adult ratio of 30:2 for all ages, including children, to simplify the algorithm and enhance memory retention.

5.3 Pulseless electrical activity (PEA): C E

This is a non-shockable rhythm. The rhythm on the monitor usually looks like sinus rhythm, but there is no pulse or signs of circulation. There have usually been signs of clinical deterioration before the event, such as worsening shock from hypovolaemia, and so many PEA arrests should be avoidable by early recognition and prompt resuscitation of the sick or injured child. PEA may be seen in hypovolaemia or in a child with a pulmonary embolus. During an arrest, it is important to consider and treat reversible causes of a cardiac arrest. These include the '4 Hs and 4 Ts': hypoxia, hypothermia, hypovolaemia and hyperkalaemia (or other metabolic disturbance, including hypokalaemia); tension pneumothorax, tamponade, toxins and thromboembolism.

5.4   Choking: B E

The initial step of the treatment algorithm is to assess the severity and whether there is an effective cough present. If the cough is effective, coughing should be encouraged. Chest thrusts are recommended in infants, because abdominal thrusts or the Heimlich manoeuvre can result in abdominal injury. Thrusts or back blows should be performed at a rate of 1 per second. A blind finger sweep is not recommended, but in the arrested child objects may be removed from the mouth under direct vision.

5.5   Hypothermia: B D E

In severe hypothermia, the heart will usually be resistant to shocks using the defibrillator and to drug therapy with adrenaline. In ventricular fibrillation, it is therefore recommended that repeated shocks are avoided. Three shocks at 4 J/kg may be attempted. Coagulation is often deranged in hypothermia, and can worsen bleeding. Rewarming frostbite can be very painful, and so analgesia is recommended. During rewarming, the peripheral vasculature dilates and results in a relative hypovolaemia, and so fluid resuscitation is usually necessary. As the metabolic needs of the body, and hence the demands placed on the heart, increase with increasing body temperature, myocardial dysfunction may only become apparent on rewarming.

5.6   Electrocution injury: A B D E

If an electrocution injury has occurred out of the home, it is usually associated with other injuries. Lightning injury is a large current of short duration, so burns, if they occur, are minor. The main injuries are either neurological, cardiac (as the current can depolarise the myocardium), or autonomic instability. If the event is unwitnessed, it is difficult to diagnose. There are often injuries from falling associated with lightning injury. Compartment syndrome is a recognised complication, and dysrhythmias can occur late. Fluid and blood have the least resistance to electricity.

5.7   Brainstem testing: B C E

Two sets of brainstem tests must be carried out with a time interval between them, by two separate doctors who are 5 years or more post-qualification. Death is pronounced after the second set of tests are completed, but the recorded time of death is at completion of the first set of testing. Oculovestibular reflexes play an important part of the brainstem testing. The doctor should first check that the ears are clear; ice-cold water is then infused into each ear over at least 60 seconds. Usually, there would be movement of the eyes towards the side on which the water is being infused. Brainstem testing is not appropriate for premature babies to confirm brainstem death, as their reflexes are not sufficiently developed.

Best of Five Answers

5.8   D: Alkalinising the urine reduces the amount of resorption in the renal tubule

Myoglobinuria occurs after muscle injury such as a crush injury or electrocution. It can be detected in the urine. The treatment involves maintaining a good urine output of greater than 2 mL/kg per hour by fluid loading and diuretics – usually mannitol – to promote an osmotic diuresis. In addition, alkalinising the urine using sodium bicarbonate infusion improves the excretion of myoglobin and keeps the toxin in its ionised form, reducing the amount of absorption in the renal tubule.

5.9   C: Airway resistance is inversely proportional to the radius to the power of 4

The upper and lower airways are smaller in children than they are in adults. As airway resistance is inversely proportional to the radius to the power of 4, a small reduction in airway size can dramatically increase the resistance in flow, resulting in airway obstruction. Halving the radius of the tube through which a gas must flow increases the resistance to the flow of gas 16-fold.

5.10 A: 8% partial thickness burn to leg

An 8% partial-thickness burn in a child does not merit referral to a burns unit. The current Advanced Paediatric Life Support (APLS) guidelines recommend the following indications for referral to a burns unit:

- a 10% or more partial-thickness burn
- a 10% burn that is a combination of partial- and full-thickness burn, even when the full-thickness component is less than 5%
- a full-thickness burn of 5% or more
- a burn to a special area such as perineum or hands, face or feet
- circumferential burn
- a significant inhalation burn
- a chemical, high-voltage or radiation burn.

5.11 D: Hyperventilation aiming for a PCO_2 between 3 and 3.5 kPa

This is no longer recommended as a neuroprotective treatment following head injury. Hyperventilation below a $PaCO_2$ of 4 kPa has been shown to result in brain ischaemia, which results in further injury following a severe head injury. Hyperventilation is only occasionally used as a temporary measure to prevent acute impending coning (APLS guidelines). The head is raised 20–30 degrees and kept in the midline, to improve venous drainage from the head. Tight control of glucose and relative hypernatraemia have also been shown to reduce the intracranial pressure and improve outcome following head injury. Avoiding both hypoxia and hypotension are important in improving outcome following brain injury.

5.12 C: Suppresses endogenous release of nitric oxide from the respiratory mucosa

Nitric oxide binds to the haem iron of guanylate cyclase, stimulating the production of cyclic guanosine monophosphate (cGMP). When given as a gas, it has marked selective pulmonary vascular effects. It has clear benefits in neonates and other patients with severe pulmonary hypertension, but may not be of benefit in the absence of pulmonary hypertension. Tolerance develops rapidly.

5.13 C: The mortality of severe sepsis in adults is three times that in children

In the USA, survival in severe sepsis was three times better in children than adults. Neonates aged less than 28 days experience the highest incidence of sepsis, at 3.6 per 1000 population. The hospital mortality is around 10%. Among children with sepsis, 49% have an underlying disease. Cardiac failure is the most common cause of death in sepsis.

EMQ Answers

5.14 Airway obstruction

1. B: Epiglottitis

The factors that influence diagnosis are the suddenness of onset, and that the child appears toxic with a very high temperature. The child can often be quiet, with minimal stridor, and unable to swallow their secretions. The vaccination history is relevant, as epiglottitis is often caused by *Haemophilus influenzae*, and the incidence has reduced since the introduction of the *H. influenzae* type B (HIB) vaccine. On tracheal intubation, the classic finding is of a cherry-red epiglottis. It can be difficult to see the vocal cords, so an experienced anaesthetist should be present. It is not always easy to differentiate clinically between epiglottitis, bacterial tracheitis and severe croup. In croup the child often looks well, and the history is usually longer.

2. E: Mediastinal tumour

The widened mediastinum indicates a mediastinal tumour causing airway obstruction. It is often confused with asthma, but a chest X-ray should be taken in a child of this age group with no previous history of asthma and an unusual presentation of airway obstruction. There is often an inspiratory component to the wheeze, which, coupled with no history of asthma, should alert the doctor to the diagnosis.

3. K: Tracheobronchomalacia

There is an association between tracheobronchomalacia and a number of cardiac abnormalities. The examination finding of a prolonged expiratory phase should alert the clinician to the possibility of this diagnosis. The clinical suspicion is confirmed by a bronchoscopy. The symptoms are worse when the child is distressed, and improve with the addition of a positive end-expiratory pressure (PEEP). As the child grows the symptoms improve, although this can take up to 2 years. Children with severe tracheobronchomalacia may need a tracheostomy to deliver PEEP.

5.15 Adrenaline (epinephrine)

Adrenaline is an inotrope which acts on β_1- and β_2-receptors, and on α-receptors.

1. C: 5 mL of 1 in 1000 adrenaline via a nebuliser

In croup, adrenaline is given via a nebuliser and acts as a β_2-agonist, causing bronchodilatation. It can also be given via this route when there is airway swelling following extubation. The dose is 5 mL of 1 in 1000 adrenaline.

2. L: 0.3 mL of 1 in 1000 adrenaline intramuscularly

In anaphylaxis, the dose of adrenaline should be given intramuscularly, as this is not a situation of arrest and in inexperienced hands intravenous adrenaline is dangerous. The concentrated dose of 1/1,000 is preferred to reduce the volume of fluid injected into the muscle. The APLS guidelines for the dose have recently changed from 0.01 mL/kg of 1/1,000 adrenaline intramuscularly to an age-related dose. The dose for an 8-year-old is 0.3 mL of 1/1,000 intramuscularly.

For children over 12 years, the adult dose is used, ie. 500 μg or 0.5 mL of 1/1,000, for 6- to 12-year-olds the dose is 0.3 mL and for children less than 6 years, the dose is 0.15 mL.

3. H: 0.1 mL/kg of 1 in 10 000 adrenaline intravenously before the third shock

In ventricular fibrillation, the dose of adrenaline is 0.1 mL/kg intravenously. This is given before the third shock, and then every 3–5 minutes until sinus rhythm returns. Amiodarone is given before the fourth shock at a dose of 5 mg/kg.

The information in this chapter is consistent with the resuscitation guidelines from APLS.

6. Endocrinology

Multiple True–False Questions

6.1   The following is true regarding tall stature in childhood:

☐ A the most common endocrine cause is a growth hormone-secreting pituitary tumour

☐ B it is associated with congenital adrenal hyperplasia

☐ C Sotos syndrome is associated with hemihypertrophy

☐ D children with karyotype 47,XYY have Klinefelter syndrome

☐ E it is associated with cystinuria

6.2   The following is true about growth hormone:

☐ A in short children, a history of chronic renal failure is a licensed indication for the use of recombinant growth hormone in the UK

☐ B recombinant human growth hormone is primarily used in Prader–Willi syndrome to improve final height

☐ C growth hormone is also known as insulin-like growth factor 1 (IGF-1)

☐ D slipped upper femoral epiphysis is a side-effect of the administration of recombinant growth hormone

☐ E the major cause of short stature in Turner syndrome is growth hormone deficiency

6.3   The following are features of Noonan syndrome:

☐ A cubitus valgus

☐ B hypertelorism

☐ C pulmonary valve stenosis

☐ D increased risk of malignancy

☐ E short 4th/5th metacarpals

6.4   The following are features associated with polycystic ovary syndrome (PCOS) in adolescence:

☐ A delayed puberty

☐ B hirsutism

☐ C hyperinsulinaemia

☐ D increased luteinising hormone (LH)

☐ E low testosterone

6.5   Pseudohypoparathyroidism type 1a is associated with

- ☐ A hypocalcaemia
- ☐ B normal stature
- ☐ C hyperphosphataemia
- ☐ D increased parathyroid hormone (PTH)
- ☐ E clinodactyly

6.6   The following can be features of multiple endocrine neoplasia (MEN) syndrome type 2a in children:

- ☐ A phaeochromocytoma
- ☐ B pituitary tumour
- ☐ C medullary thyroid carcinoma
- ☐ D hyperparathyroidism
- ☐ E gastrinoma

6.7   The following hormones are secreted by the anterior pituitary gland:

- ☐ A growth hormone
- ☐ B gonadotrophin-releasing hormone
- ☐ C adrenocorticotrophic hormone
- ☐ D prolactin
- ☐ E vasopressin

6.8   Cushing syndrome

- ☐ A in childhood is usually secondary to pituitary tumours
- ☐ B commonly results in obese, tall children
- ☐ C is normally straightforward to diagnose in childhood
- ☐ D when secondary to Cushing's disease, has been caused by adrenal pathology
- ☐ E that is associated with a low adrenocorticotrophic hormone (ACTH) and failure to suppress cortisol with high-dose dexamethasone is likely to be due to an adrenal tumour

Best of Five Questions

6.9   Thyroid hormone resistance is BEST characterised by:

- ☐ A   High T$_3$, high T$_4$, low thyroid-stimulating hormone (TSH)
- ☐ B   Low T$_3$, low T$_4$, low TSH
- ☐ C   Low T$_3$, low T$_4$, high TSH
- ☐ D   High T$_3$, high T$_4$, normal TSH
- ☐ E   Normal T$_3$, normal T$_4$, high TSH

6.10 A 6-year-old girl presents with a 6-week history of bone pain, increased thirst, polyuria, weight loss, lethargy and abdominal pain. Examination shows a thin girl with mild dehydration. The abdomen is soft with no organomegaly. Investigations show sodium 147 mmol/L, potassium 3.8 mmol/L, urea 8.1 mmol/L, creatinine 90 μmol/L, phosphate 1.6 mmol/L, corrected calcium 3.95 mmol/L, alkaline phosphatase (ALP) 65 IU/L (normal range 69–325 IU/L), albumin 35 g/L, parathyroid hormone (PTH) < 0.1 pg/ml. What is the MOST likely diagnosis?

- ☐ A   Pseudohypoparathyroidism
- ☐ B   Parathyroid adenoma
- ☐ C   Acute lymphoblastic leukaemia
- ☐ D   Renal osteodystrophy
- ☐ E   Familial benign hypercalcaemia

6.11 A 5-year-old girl presents with short stature. She has always been short, but this has become more apparent over the past year. Her height is below the 2nd centile, and her weight is on the 2nd centile. She is asymptomatic. She is not dysmorphic. What would the MOST useful investigation be?

- ☐ A   Thyroid function tests
- ☐ B   Chromosomes
- ☐ C   Coeliac screen
- ☐ D   Full blood count
- ☐ E   C-reactive protein

6.12 A 13-year-old girl presents to clinic with a 1-year history of abdominal pain. She has been finding games lessons at school very tiring, but has been managing a full day at school without any problems. Her school work has remained at the same high standard. Her mother has noticed that her shoe size has not changed over the past 2 years. Examination revealed: weight 75th centile, height 25th centile; rounded face, not flushed; pulse 60 beats/min, blood pressure 100/60 mmHg; abdomen had palpable faeces; breast stage 3; pubic/axillary hair stage 1. What is the MOST likely diagnosis?

☐ A   Addison's disease
☐ B   Cushing syndrome
☐ C   Hypothyroidism
☐ D   Chronic fatigue syndrome
☐ E   Constitutional delay of growth and puberty

6.13 On the postnatal ward you review a baby 36 hours of age. Ambiguous genitalia have been noted on the baby check. Examination reveals: the baby has a phallus 1.8 cm long with a urethral opening at the distal end; the genital folds are fused midline; there are no palpable gonads. Which investigation would be MOST informative at this time?

☐ A   Ultrasound scan of the pelvis
☐ B   17-Hydroxyprogesterone (17-OHP)
☐ C   Urea and electrolytes (U&E)
☐ D   Inhibin B
☐ E   Human chorionic gonadotrophin (hCG) test

Extended Matching Questions

6.14 Theme: Puberty

A   21-Hydroxylase deficiency
B   Central precocious puberty
C   Ovarian insufficiency
D   Premature thelarche
E   Complete androgen insensitivity syndrome
F   Hypothyroidism
G   Gonadal tumour
H   Hypogonadotrophic hypogonadism
I   Hypopituitarism
J   McCune–Albright syndrome

For each of the scenarios below, select the matching option from the above list. Each option may be used once, more than once, or not at all.

☐   1.   A 1-year-old girl presents with a 6-month history of breast development bilaterally. Growth, bone age and pelvic ultrasound are normal for her age. A luteinising hormone-releasing hormone (LHRH) stimulation test shows an exaggerated follicle-stimulating hormone (FSH) response, but with a prepubertal LH response. Examination shows Tanner stage B2, PH1, A1.

☐   2.   A 14-year-old girl has a previous history of unilateral Wilms tumour treated with abdominal irradiation and cyclophosphamide. She is pre-menarchal. Examination showed she was 50th centile for height and weight, with a recent increase in height velocity. Pubertal staging was Tanner stage B2, P2, A2. Investigations demonstrated a basal FSH of 28 U/L (normal range 3–8 U/L), LH 20 U/L (normal range 2–8 U/L), and oestradiol 100 pmol/L. Bone age was 13 years 6 months.

☐   3.   A 6-year-old boy presents with acne, pubic and axillary hair development, penis enlargement and mood swings. Serial height measurements demonstrate an increase in height velocity. He has a bone age advanced by 2 years and examination reveals pubertal stage PH2, G2 with 2-mL testes bilaterally.

6.15 Theme: Basic science of hormones

A   Cortisol
B   Thyroxine (or thyroid hormone)
C   Testosterone
D   Growth hormone
E   Insulin
F   Glucagon
G   Luteinising hormone
H   Aldosterone
I   Follicle-stimulating hormone
J   Oestrogen

For each of the scenarios below, select the hormone that is most likely to act in this way. Each option may be used once, more than once, or not at all.

☐ 1. This hormone has a continuous pattern of secretion and is regulated by a hormone produced by the pituitary gland.

☐ 2. This hormone has a pulsatile pattern of secretion. In the male, it binds to the Leydig cells, which stimulate the first step in testosterone production.

☐ 3. Adrenocorticotrophic hormone (ACTH) causes a temporary increase in this hormone, although the effect is not sustained. The hormone is secreted from the zona glomerulosa of the adrenal cortex.

MT–F Answers

6.1 Tall stature in childhood: B

Familial tall stature is by far the most common cause of tall stature, and shows a normal height velocity. The androgen excess of untreated congenital adrenal hyperplasia leads to tall stature in childhood but, ultimately, short stature in adulthood. The most common endocrinopathies that cause tall stature are precocious puberty and hyperthyroidism. A growth hormone-secreting tumour is a very rare cause of tall stature in childhood. Sotos syndrome is a pre- and postnatal overgrowth syndrome with normal growth hormone secretion. Features include increased birth weight, length and head circumference. Affected individuals have hypotonia, clumsiness, a large elongated forehead, and learning difficulties. Rapid growth occurs in early childhood and is associated with an advanced bone age. There is a slightly early puberty and a final adult height in the upper part of the normal range. Hemihypertrophy occurs in Beckwith–Wiedemann syndrome. The karyotype of Klinefelter syndrome has additional X chromosomes; the karyotype is usually 47,XXY, but can be XXXY. This occurs as a result of maternal or paternal non-dysjunction during the first meiotic division. Cystinuria is a disorder of transport of cystine (amino acids) – cystine is insoluble in urine and patients develop renal calculi. There is no association with tall stature. Homocystinuria is an autosomal recessive condition affecting amino acid metabolism (cystathionine β-synthetase deficiency). The physical appearance is similar to Marfan syndrome, and clinical features include downward lens dislocation, tall stature, and mental retardation. There is increased risk of thromboembolic events and osteoporosis.

6.2 Growth hormone: A D

Adequate release of growth hormone (GH) is a major factor responsible for normal linear growth in childhood, whereas nutrition is the major factor in infancy. For the treatment of short stature in childhood, licensed indications for recombinant human growth hormone (rhGH) in the UK are growth hormone deficiency, Turner syndrome, chronic renal failure, and children born small for gestational age. The side-effects of rhGH administration include benign intracranial hypertension, slipped upper femoral epiphysis, glucose intolerance and scoliosis. Hypothyroidism can also be unmasked. Previous concerns regarding an association between rhGH administration and childhood leukaemia have been refuted by a number of epidemiological studies. For children with Prader–Willi syndrome, rhGH is primarily used to improve body composition and tone.

GH is produced in the somatotrophs in the anterior pituitary and binds to GH target-organ receptors, primarily in liver. This induces synthesis of insulin-like growth factor 1 (IGF-1). IGF-1 enters the circulation bound to specific carrier proteins called IGF-binding proteins. IGF-1 is delivered to its IGF-1 receptor at a target site, eg the growth plate of a long bone, where it stimulates longitudinal growth. GH improves bone mineral density and lean mass, and maintains normal lipid composition. Short stature in Turner syndrome is mostly accounted for by a defect in a short stature homeobox gene (*SHOX*) in the Xp22 region. Use of rhGH is licensed in Turner syndrome, and recent studies suggest that a mean increase in final height of 6–8 cm can be expected if GH is given.

6.3 Noonan syndrome: A B C D

Noonan syndrome occurs in 1 in 1000–2500 live births, with a male:female ratio of 1:1. It can be inherited in an autosomal dominant manner, although it can occur sporadically. The phenotype is varied, but it must be considered in any child presenting with short stature. The features are: short stature, hypertelorism, ptosis, epicanthic folds, down-slanting palpebral fissures, low-set ears, webbed neck, cubitus valgus, coagulation problems, cryptorchidism, delayed puberty and mild intellectual impairment. Congenital cardiac defects occur in 60–70% of those affected; pulmonary valve stenosis is the most common. Some mutations (*PTPN 11* gene, 50%; *SOS1* gene, 13%; *KRAS* gene, 5%) are known to cause Noonan syndrome. Noonan syndrome (particularly *PTPN 11* gene abnormalities) is associated with an increased risk of developing juvenile myelomonocytic leukaemia (JMML). Shortened 4th/5th metacarpals is a feature of Turner syndrome.

6.4 Polycystic ovary syndrome in adolescents: B C D

PCOS is diagnosed with increasing frequency in females during adolescence, and consists of at least two of the following:

- polycystic ovaries
- features of hyperandrogenism, eg hirsutism
- anovulation.

There may be a previous history of premature adrenarche and early puberty. Although the exact cause is uncertain, insulin resistance may be a feature of PCOS, even in non-obese patients. The insulin resistance leads to hyperinsulinaemia as pancreatic insulin secretion increases to maintain normoglycaemia. The likelihood of insulin resistance is affected by genetic predisposition, physical activity, visceral obesity, hyperandrogenism, medications (thiazides, corticosteroids), increasing age, and pregnancy.

Investigations in PCOS will classically show:

- increased adrenal androgens (testosterone, androstenedione, dehydroepiandrosterone sulphate [DHEAS])
- low sex hormone-binding globulin
- increased LH/FSH ratio in postpubertal girls.

Women with PCOS have an increased risk of myocardial infarction, ischaemic heart disease, type 2 diabetes mellitus, and impaired glucose tolerance. Where appropriate, the primary aim of management is weight reduction. The medical treatment includes the insulin sensitiser, metformin. The oral contraceptive pill (oestrogen with or without an antiandrogen) can be used to reduce acne and hirsutism by inhibition of ovarian androgen, and to suppress LH and follicle-stimulating hormone (FSH).

6.5   Pseudohypoparathyroidism type 1a: A B C D

Pseudohypoparathyroidism type 1a is condition in which there is resistance to parathyroid hormone in a number of different tissues; it is generally inherited in autosomal dominant manner (but may also occur sporadically). Children are usually short and obese, but can also have normal stature. The clinical features include: round face, short neck, short stature, obesity, shortened 4th metacarpal and metatarsal, reduced IQ, intracranial and subcutaneous calcification, sensorineural deafness and poor sense of smell. Biochemical features include low calcium, increased phosphate and increased PTH. Clinodactyly in a short, obese child would suggest Laurence–Moon–Biedl syndrome or Prader–Willi syndrome.

6.6   Multiple endocrine neoplasia (MEN) syndrome type 2a: A C D

MEN syndromes are defined by the presence of tumours involving two or more endocrine glands. All MEN syndromes can be autosomal dominant or can occur sporadically. There is variable penetrance.

- **MEN type 1** is characterised by parathyroid, pancreatic, endocrine and anterior pituitary tumours. MEN 1 is caused by mutations in the *MENIN* gene.
- **MEN type 2a** is characterised by medullary thyroid carcinoma (MTC), phaeochromocytoma and hyperparathyroidism.
- **MEN type 2b** involves MTC, phaeochromocytoma and mucosal neuromas.

MEN 2 syndromes are due to faulty tyrosine kinase receptors caused by mutations in the *RET* proto-oncogene. In MEN 2a, genetic testing should be carried out before the child reaches the age of 5 years. For patients with *RET* mutations, prophylactic total thyroidectomy is recommended to prevent the development of medullary thyroid carcinoma. Regular biochemical monitoring is necessary from age 5 years, with annual measurement of serum calcitonin (a marker of medullary thyroid carcinoma) and 24-hour catecholamine collections (screen for phaeochromocytoma) and serum calcium and PTH from age 10 years (screen for hyperparathyroidism).

6.7   Hormones secreted by the anterior pituitary gland: A C D

The pituitary gland lies within the sella turcica at the base of the brain. The anterior pituitary gland develops from the ectoderm of the buccal mucosa and the posterior pituitary gland is derived from neural ectoderm from the diencephalon. The anterior pituitary gland secretes growth hormone, adrenocorticotrophic hormone, thyroid-stimulating hormone, luteinising hormone, follicle-stimulating hormone and prolactin. The posterior pituitary gland releases vasopressin and oxytocin. Vasopressin and oxytocin are synthesised in magnocellular neurones in supraoptic and paraventricular nuclei of the hypothalamus, and are then transported along supraoptic–hypophyseal neurones to be stored in the posterior pituitary for subsequent release. Gonadotrophin-releasing hormone is secreted by the hypothalamus into the pituitary portal circulation.

6.8   Cushing syndrome: E

Cushing syndrome is not common in childhood. The majority of cases are secondary to iatrogenic steroids given orally, by inhalation, intranasally, topically or intravenously. Other aetiologies include adrenocorticotrophic hormone (ACTH)-secreting pituitary tumours (Cushing's disease), adrenal adenoma/carcinoma, adrenal hyperplasia, and ectopic ACTH. A characteristic feature in childhood Cushing syndrome is growth arrest. Simple obesity is associated with normal or advanced growth. The diagnosis of Cushing syndrome in children is often difficult; this is because of the pulsatile nature in which the relevant hormones are secreted: 24-hour urinary free cortisol levels can appear normal on the first two collections and then show gross elevation when repeated 1 month later. Initial investigations include at least two 24-hour urinary free cortisol measurements, 0800 h and midnight (while sleeping) cortisol and ACTH, to look for loss of normal diurnal variation, and dexamethasone suppression tests. Cushing syndrome with a low ACTH and failure to suppress cortisol with high-dose dexamethasone is likely to be secondary to adrenal pathology. A high ACTH and some cortisol and ACTH suppression with high-dose dexamethasone may be due to a pituitary abnormality. A high ACTH that does not suppress with high-dose dexamethasone may be secondary to ectopic ACTH, which is extremely rare in childhood. However, the aetiology is rarely so clear-cut, and often the secreting tumours are difficult to pick up, even with high-resolution MRI.

Best of Five Answers

6.9   D: High T_3, high T_4, normal TSH

Answer A is thyrotoxicosis. Answer B is suggestive of secondary or central hypothyroidism. Answer C is primary hypothyroidism. Answer E is compensated hypothyroidism (in primary hypothyroidism the TSH is increased) – the thyroxine can be low (overt hypothyroidism) or normal (compensated hypothyroidism). Thyroid hormone resistance is a rare autosomal dominant disorder characterised by increased free T_4 and T_3, with an inappropriate normal or high TSH. It is due to a mutation in the TRβ subunit of the thyroid hormone receptor. There may be variable tissue resistance to thyroxine throughout the body. The presentation is variable, and thyroid hormone resistance is often diagnosed incidentally when thyroid function is checked because of non-specific signs.

6.10 C: Acute lymphoblastic leukaemia

The results show increased calcium with suppressed parathyroid hormone (PTH) and normal phosphate. The clinical features are typical of hypercalcaemia. In children presenting with hypercalcaemia, it is important to consider malignancy. Hypercalcaemia in childhood malignancy may be caused by direct invasion of the tumour into bone or by release of factors that promote osteoclastic bone resorption. Parathyroid hormone-related peptide (PTHrP) may also be released by some tumours and contribute to hypercalcaemia (PTHrP has bone effects similar to those of PTH). The ALP is inappropriately low for this age, suggesting there is a low bone turnover state – ie inhibition of bone turnover.

Pseudohypoparathyroidism shows low calcium, increased PTH and increased phosphate as a result of peripheral resistance to the actions of PTH. Parathyroid adenomas are very rare in childhood. They result in primary hyperparathyroidism, which will cause raised PTH, low phosphate and high calcium. Renal osteodystrophy describes secondary hyperparathyroidism in chronic renal failure and shows low calcium, raised phosphate and low/normal PTH. Familial benign hypercalcaemia features increased plasma calcium throughout life, with an inappropriately normal PTH. This is autosomal dominant, and is caused by defects in the calcium-sensing receptor.

6.11 B: Chromosomes

Turner syndrome is caused by complete or partial absence of one of the X chromosomes in a female. It must always be excluded in any female presenting with short stature. The incidence is 1 in 2500 live-born girls.

There may not be any apparent dysmorphic features, and it has been diagnosed late in adult women presenting to gynaecological clinics with difficulty conceiving.

The possible dysmorphic features include:

- pedal oedema
- low hairline
- neck webbing
- high-arched palate
- café-au-lait spots
- cubitus valgus

- hyper-convex nails
- widely spaced nipples
- shield-shaped chest
- short 4th and 5th metacarpals
- associated cardiac defects (eg coarctation)
- renal anomalies (eg horseshoe kidney).

Up to 20% of girls can spontaneously enter puberty and may achieve menses, but the majority require oestrogen therapy. Those who have spontaneous puberty should be warned that it does not mean they will produce ova. There are now many women with Turner syndrome who have had a pregnancy following in-vitro fertilisation (IVF) with a donor egg. In view of this, it is essential to introduce oestrogen therapy gradually, to ensure adequate breast and uterine development. These girls need to be followed up and investigated for possible thyroid problems, middle-ear disease, hypertension and insulin resistance. Learning difficulties can occur, particularly in maths. Hypothyroidism does result in short stature, but children with short stature as a result of hypothyroidism are usually overweight. Coeliac disease in young children often presents with symptoms, but can be asymptomatic, with poor growth as a manifestation. Full blood count and C-reactive protein may be abnormal, but are unlikely in this case to lead to a specific diagnosis.

6.12 C: Hypothyroidism

Acquired hypothyroidism usually has an insidious onset. There is often weight gain and reduced height velocity. Lack of energy, cold intolerance, constipation, and dry skin and hair are also presenting features. Most children will change shoe size once or twice a year if they have a normal growth velocity; often parents are more aware of changes in shoe size than change in height. Very high levels of thyroid-stimulating hormone (TSH) may cross-react with follicle-stimulating hormone (FSH) receptors and stimulate the release of oestradiol from the ovaries, leading to breast development. School performance usually remains normal.

Addison's disease is associated with poor weight gain and hypotension. Cushing syndrome is associated with androgenisation secondary to over-stimulation of the adrenal glands, hypertension and plethoric facies.

Chronic fatigue syndrome commonly results in poor school attendance; it is not associated with decreased growth, but may be associated with increased weight gain secondary to inactivity. Constitutional delay of growth and puberty can result in delayed puberty, and poor weight and height gain. Girls who are overweight tend to enter puberty early rather than late, and have associated pubic hair following initial breast development.

6.13 A: Ultrasound scan of the pelvis

This can be a very complex condition to deal with, and it is important to liaise early with local specialists – ie paediatric endocrinologists and paediatric urologists. It is imperative to perform karyotype testing as quickly as possible (the results take 24–56 hours to process). It is important to explain to the parents that the chromosomal sex is not necessarily the most important determining factor in deciding the sex of rearing. An ultrasound scan of the pelvis will give the most immediate information as to what the diagnosis might be. It will be possible to tell if there are internal female genitalia (müllerian structures), and you can also look for undescended testes. The presence of a uterus indicates the absence of testicular tissue or failure of testicular tissue to synthesise anti-müllerian hormone.

17-Hydroxyprogesterone is very important and needs to be measured to rule out congenital adrenal hyperplasia (CAH). All babies have increased 17-OHP after delivery, and the level is best measured 48 hours after birth to avoid falsely high results. Most laboratories will be unable to give a result on the day when the sample is taken. U&E will be normal at day 2, even if the diagnosis is CAH. Babies who present with a collapse secondary to CAH usually present on about day 10 with a salt-losing crisis. Inhibin B is produced by Sertoli cells and acts to suppress FSH activity. An undetectable value suggests anorchia, so is a helpful test in investigation of an XY infant with no palpable gonads. The hCG stimulation test is used to detect functioning testicular tissue and define enzyme blocks in testosterone biosynthesis. If required, the test can be performed at a later date.

EMQ Answers

6.14 Puberty

1. D: Premature thelarche

Premature thelarche describes benign isolated breast development, which can be unilateral or bilateral. It most often occurs between the ages of 6 months and 2 years. Growth, bone age, and pelvic ultrasound are consistent with chronological age. Endocrine investigations may show FSH secretion and some ovarian function greater than prepubertal controls. At breast stage 3, central precocious puberty would typically present with development of pubic and axillary hair, increased height velocity, and pubertal change on pelvic ultrasound scan. Gonadal tumours are rare, as is McCune–Albright syndrome, but both could present with isolated breast development. However, in these latter conditions the increased sex steroids produced would cause oestrogen-mediated changes in the uterus, leading to pubertal changes on ultrasound, with or without menstruation.

2. C: Ovarian insufficiency

This girl has pubertal arrest, with delayed menarche and increased gonadotrophins. These results suggest that the hypothalamic–pituitary axis is functioning and is trying to hyperstimulate the failing ovaries. Gonadal dysfunction after oncology treatment can be due to irradiation or gonadotoxic chemotherapy. Cyclophosphamide is a well-known cause of gonadal failure. The girl has produced detectable oestradiol, indicating that her gonads have not completely failed, and that she has ovarian insufficiency rather than complete gonadal failure. She is likely to require treatment (oestrogen) to assist progression through puberty and is likely to have fertility problems.

3. A: 21-Hydroxylase deficiency

This boy has symptoms and signs of androgen excess: acne, penile enlargement, and pubic and axillary hair. Central precocious puberty or a gonadal tumour could cause his increased height velocity, but the former would cause bilateral testicular enlargement and the latter unilateral (with contralateral testicular atrophy). Non-classic (ie non-salt-wasting) congenital adrenal hyperplasia can present in childhood with signs of androgen excess. The most common would be simple virilising 21-hydroxylase deficiency.

6.15 Basic science of hormones

1. **B: Thyroid hormone**
2. **G: Luteinising hormone**
3. **H: Aldosterone**

Hormones are chemical messengers produced by a variety of specialised cells. There are three main types of hormones: amine, steroid and peptide. Hormones may be secreted in a continuous pattern (eg thyroxine) or an intermittent pattern (FSH, LH, GH, prolactin, cortisol, ACTH). The hormones secreted by the anterior pituitary gland are luteinising hormone (LH), follicle-stimulating hormone (FSH), growth hormone, adrenocorticotrophic hormone (ACTH) and thyroid-stimulating hormone (TSH). In the male, LH binds to Leydig cells and stimulates the first step in testosterone production. In the female it binds to ovarian cells and stimulates steroidogenesis. FSH binds to the Sertoli cells in the male and increases the mass of the seminiferous tubules and supports the development of sperm. In the female, FSH binds to the glomerulosa cells and stimulates the conversion of testosterone to oestrogen. Growth hormone has a pulsatile secretion pattern consisting of peaks and troughs, and acts via the second messenger of insulin-like growth factor 1 (IGF-1). TSH is a trophic hormone and causes the release and production of thyroid hormone, T_4. ACTH is responsible for stimulation of the adrenal cortex, and in particular the production of cortisol. It produces a temporary rise in aldosterone, but this is not sustained. Aldosterone is primarily regulated by the renin–angiotensin system in response to electrolyte balance and plasma volumes. The adrenal cortex has three principal functions: glucocorticoid production (cortisol) in the zona fasciculata; mineralocorticoid production (aldosterone) in the zona glomerulosa; androgen production (testosterone, dehydroepiandrosterone sulphate [DHEAS]) in the zona reticularis.

7. Ethics, Law and Governance

Multiple True–False Questions

7.1   The moral duties of doctors include:

☐   A   offering treatments that carry more benefits than harms
☐   B   always following the wishes of parents because this respects their right to make choices for their child
☐   C   respecting the human dignity of children who are able to express their views
☐   D   obtaining written consent for medical interventions
☐   E   providing personal information about patients when requested to do so by anyone

7.2   Which of the following are true of the duty of confidentiality?

☐   A   consent for disclosure of personal information should always be sought
☐   B   information must be disclosed if a court requests it
☐   C   when sharing information, only the minimum necessary for the intended purpose should be given
☐   D   anonymised information should always be used
☐   E   information may be freely shared within healthcare teams providing care for a child, unless the parents object

7.3   Contraception may be legally provided to a 15-year-old girl without parental consent or knowledge if

☐   A   she demands it because she is frightened to say 'No' to her boyfriend
☐   B   she refuses to discuss matters with her parents, reminding you that she has refused to do so before
☐   C   a low-dose oestrogen pill is used
☐   D   she understands the implication of contraception for herself and her family
☐   E   her parents are abroad

7.4 Abortion is legal in children under the age of 16 years if

☐ A a single doctor assesses the child

☐ B the child is able to understand what is involved and its likely consequences

☐ C there is a substantial risk that the child to be born will be seriously handicapped

☐ D continuing the pregnancy would be likely to damage the physical and mental health of the child's father

☐ E the pregnancy does not exceed 28 weeks

7.5 Parental responsibility

☐ A is automatically acquired by the woman who gives birth to the baby

☐ B is transferred to the local authority as a result of a Care Order

☐ C is lost by the birth mother if her baby is adopted

☐ D is lost by the mother when the child reaches majority

☐ E is lost by the mother when the child becomes able to make their own decisions

7.6 The capacity for a child to consent for treatment

☐ A is recognised by Act of Parliament in a 16-year-old

☐ B requires court approval if they are younger than 16 years

☐ C is considered with equal weight for assent or refusal at 15 years

☐ D was challenged by Gillick & Sons (Solicitors) in 1983

☐ E is not accepted below the age of 12 years

7.7 The following can legally refuse consent to treatment in the following circumstances:

☐ A a 14-year-old Fraser ruling (Gillick)-competent boy with leukaemia who requires blood transfusions but objects on religious grounds

☐ B the parents of a 2-year-old boy with leukaemia in relapse after bone marrow transplant

☐ C the parents of a baby born alive at 23 weeks' gestation

☐ D the parents of a baby with Down syndrome and duodenal atresia

☐ E the mother of a 15-year-old girl who has requested termination of pregnancy

7.8   The following statements are compatible with the application of utilitarian moral theories:

☐ A   the reasonably foreseeable consequences of an action determine its rightness or wrongness

☐ B   children should have special provision in terms of healthcare

☐ C   withdrawal of life-sustaining treatment from an extremely sick premature infant is justified, even if parents object

☐ D   vaccination programmes that secure herd immunity at the expense of some side-effects are morally justified

☐ E   they provide clear answers as to what action individuals should choose

7.9   The following are true with respect to children's rights:

☐ A   the United Nations Convention on the Rights of the Child forms part of the law of the UK

☐ B   a child who is capable of forming their views should be allowed to express them

☐ C   all children have an absolute right to life-sustaining treatment

☐ D   the UK Human Rights Act (UKHRA) makes specific provision for children

☐ E   children may defer decision-making to others, even if they are capable of making their own choices

Best of Five Questions

7.10 In casualty, you see a baby of 4 months with bruises on its arm. Mum says the baby fell out of its cot. You also notice old bruising, and an X-ray shows a spiral fracture of the humerus. It is 2000 h, there is no social worker in the hospital, and the baby is not on the protection register. What do you do?

☐ A   Ask for an orthopaedic opinion and send the baby home

☐ B   Tell mum she needs to wait for blood results in casualty

☐ C   Tell mum she needs to wait until a skeletal survey is done

☐ D   Tell mum she needs to wait until social services speak to her

☐ E   Admit child to the ward, observe and investigate further

7.11 It is 1700 h, and you are asked to see a 15-year-old girl who has been admitted with a new diagnosis of leukaemia. Her heart rate is 120 beats/min, she has a gallop rhythm and a soft murmur. Her haemoglobin is 6.5 g/dL. Because of their religious beliefs, the parents are refusing a blood transfusion. The girl also refuses. What do you do?

- [ ] A Start chemotherapy but do not give transfusion
- [ ] B Ask for a Police Protection Order
- [ ] C Give the blood transfusion
- [ ] D Ask for a Court Order before giving the transfusion
- [ ] E Ask for psychiatric assessment of the girl, to assess her decision-making capacity

7.12 Jim is 14 and in early puberty. He has developed a non-Hodgkin's lymphoma (NHL) and will receive chemotherapy, which is highly likely to impair his future fertility. His parents are anxious that something is done because they believe that he will want children in the future. What is the MOST appropriate intervention?

- [ ] A Reassure the family that Jim will be fine
- [ ] B Ask Jim to provide a sample of sperm for banking
- [ ] C Arrange for Jim to have an assessment of his capacity to consent to treatment
- [ ] D Arrange for Jim to have a testicular biopsy to collect gametes
- [ ] E Proceed with sperm banking, with parental consent

7.13 Legal consent for the ritual circumcision of a 12-year-old boy is BEST obtained in which way?

- [ ] A From the biological mother
- [ ] B From both parents
- [ ] C Over the telephone
- [ ] D From the boy if he is Gillick competent
- [ ] E Orally, rather than in writing

Extended Matching Questions

7.14 Theme: Consent

A   Family solicitor
B   Family doctor
C   Aunt
D   Stepmother
E   Genetic mother
F   Biological father
G   Parent with parental responsibility
H   Twin brother

For each of the following, which person from the list above is best identified? Each option may be used once, more than once, or not at all.

☐   1.   In the absence of a order issued or ratified by the Family Court, the most likely person who can give consent for a 3-year-old needing heart surgery.
☐   2.   Among those listed who do not have automatic rights to parental responsibility, the most likely person to have it.

7.15 Theme: Capacity

A   Person with Gillick competence
B   Person with presumed competence
C   Person aged 18 years
D   Person aged 15 years
E   A 17-year-old Jehovah's Witness
F   Person aged 21 years
G   Person aged 11 years
H   A mother of any age

From the above list, select the youngest person described in the following situations:

☐   1.   Can enforce refusal of a life-saving blood transfusion.
☐   2.   Can give sole consent for an appendectomy.

MT–F Answers

7.1 Moral duties of doctors: A

The moral duty of doctors to act in the best interests of their patients is a fundamental principle that underpins contemporary medical practice. It involves offering treatments that are intended to provide net benefits over harms. In this context, harms may be physical, psychological or social. Although parents do have ethical and legal authority to decide for their child, they may do so only if they act in the child's best interests. Sometimes their choices and preferences (eg the use of experimental or unproven treatments) may not be in the child's best interests. Paediatricians should respect the human dignity of children regardless of their ability to express their views. To do otherwise would be to discriminate against the weak and vulnerable. Although all medical interventions require consent of the patient or those with the legal authority to consent on their behalf, this does not have to be written. The circumstances in which it is felt necessary to obtain written or witnessed consent are a matter of professional judgement, but are likely to include complex or controversial procedures or situations in which professionals feel that there may be a future legal action. Personal information can be provided if there is consent to do so, or if it is essential to share information amongst members of a team to provide treatment that is in the best interests of the child. Older children may consent to sharing of information if they have the capacity to do so. Information should not otherwise be routinely provided to all who request it unless those who do so have clear legal authority or there is a clear public interest obligation to do so.

7.2 Duty of confidentiality: B C E

There is a general professional duty of confidentiality that applies just as much to children as it does to adults. In general, personal information should not be disclosed without the consent of the patient – or, in the case of children, those with parental responsibility – but this is not absolute. There may be circumstances in which it is necessary to share information in order to prevent significant harm to children, irrespective of consent, but the person who discloses information needs to justify their actions. Disclosure of information is a legal duty in certain circumstances, eg notification of certain specified infectious diseases, notification of births and deaths, or if the court makes a specific request for it. There is a general expectation that information will be shared amongst members of a healthcare team so that effective treatment that is in the child's best interests can be given. All members of the team should understand and respect their corporate and individual duty of confidentiality. However, parental objections should be honoured, unless to do so places the child at risk of significant harm. When considering how much information to share, a certain amount of professional discretion and judgement are necessary, but in general the amount shared should be the minimum judged necessary to accomplish the intended purpose. In some circumstances it is good practice to use anonymised data, eg when ascertaining the prevalence of certain conditions for public health purposes. However, this may not always be possible or desirable, eg in rare conditions that effectively identify the patient, or when it is necessary to do so to prevent significant harm.

7.3   Provision of contraception to a 15-year-old girl: B D

The legal criteria for prescribing contraception without parental knowledge or consent were laid down by Lord Fraser in the Gillick judgement and are referred to as Fraser's criteria. They are:

- ability to understand the implications for self and family
- a sustained and consistent refusal to discuss with parents
- the young person has made a decision to start or continue to have sexual intercourse, despite attempts at persuasion otherwise
- the adolescent's health will suffer or is likely to suffer if contraception is not given
- prescribing contraception is in the young person's best interests.

This girl has shown persistent reluctance to discuss the matter with her parents, and appears to understand fully the implications of contraception for herself and her family. Presumably, the latter would include the fact that her family may serendipitously discover the fact that she is taking contraception. The fact that the girl's parents are not in the country is not a criterion for contraception. She should be persuaded to contact them or to discuss matters with the person who is appointed to act as legal guardian in their absence. The fact that the girl is frightened of her boyfriend implies that she is not giving appropriately valid consent to sexual intercourse with him. This situation requires careful handling, and the need to prescribe a contraceptive would need to be balanced against the need to protect the girl from non-consensual sex. The law does not specify the type of contraception that should be taken, although clearly it should be one that confers maximal benefit and minimal harm, and one that is tailored to the specific needs of the girl in question. This may be a low-dose oestrogen pill, but need not be.

7.4   Abortion in children younger than 16 years: B C

The conditions under which children and young people may request termination of pregnancy are essentially those set out in the Abortion Act of 1967 as amended in 1990. In order to make a claim under the Act, the child will need to show that she is Gillick competent unless a person with parental responsibility makes an application on their behalf. As is the case for adults, two doctors are required to make an assessment. In children under the age of 16 years, one of these is likely to be a psychiatrist, whose function is to assess the child's capacity and their mental state. The criteria for offering an abortion include the substantial risk that, if the child were born, it would suffer from such physical or mental abnormalities as to be seriously handicapped. Although the physical or mental health of the mother is an important consideration, that of the father is not. It should be borne in mind that, in a number of concealed pregnancies in teenagers, there may have been sexual abuse by a member of the family. The Act also provides, as a result of the 1990 amendment, that the time limit for abortion is 24 and not 28 weeks. However, abortions later than 28 weeks can occur if the continuation of the pregnancy would involve a risk to the life of the mother greater than if it were not terminated. As the Act is likely to see further amendments, you should seek legal advice over the issue of late abortions (ie post-28 weeks), if necessary.

7.5   Parental responsibility: A C D

Parental responsibility is automatically conferred on the woman who gives birth to a baby. The child's father acquires parental responsibility provided that he is married to the mother, and his parental responsibility dates from that marriage. For babies born after 1 December 2003, an unmarried father also acquires parental responsibility if his name is registered on the birth certificate. Parental responsibility can only be transferred away from a parent by adoption. It can be shared with a local authority, but it is not transferable. The mother retains her rights and responsibilities during the period when the child is subject to a Care Order. Parental responsibility survives until the child reaches majority, although priority is often given to the views of a competent adolescent. A child's capacity for decision-making may therefore have a bearing on the extent to which that child is permitted to exercise autonomy, but this does not negate parental responsibility.

7.6   Capacity for a child to consent for treatment: A

The Family Law Reform Act 1969 conferred the right to consent to treatment on 16- and 17-year-olds, even though they have not yet reached the age of majority (18 years in the UK). Children can provide valid consent at any age if they can be shown to be competent to make the particular decision with which they are faced. Their competence ('capacity') is assessed according to the criteria established during the Victoria Gillick case. The child must therefore be able to understand the nature and need for the procedure, the risks and benefits, the consequences of not having the procedure, and the alternatives available. All these issues need to be discussed in language that the child can understand. The assessor, who will be the senior doctor taking consent, must be satisfied that the child can retain these concepts for long enough to consider them carefully, so being able to come to a firm conclusion. If the child is found to be 'Gillick competent' then no further consent from parents is required. However, it is vital that the seriousness of the proposed treatment is taken into consideration. Although 8-year-olds might have capacity to consent for a venepuncture, it is less likely that they are competent to agree to repair of an inguinal hernia. Similarly, 13-year-olds may demonstrate capacity to consent to an emergency appendectomy, but might struggle to demonstrate capacity to consent to a course of cytotoxic chemotherapy. In general terms, the Gillick doctrine is applied to assent rather than dissent. Parental responsibility is retained until the child reaches the age of 18 years, and during all of this time a parent can supply the consent that is required for treatment, even against the wishes of a Gillick-competent dissenter. Just how strongly the treatment is enforced depends on the seriousness of the illness. A child in this category may well be permitted to 'escape' treatment for a scarred foreskin if they are sufficiently determined. However, the courts will not permit a child to die of treatable disease merely because they refuse to co-operate.

7.7   Legal refusal to consent to be treated: B C

The legal ability to refuse treatment is not the corollary of the ability to consent. This is especially the case when refusal will lead to the risk of serious harm to the mental or physical health of the minor. Courts are reluctant to allow young people to take actions that will lead to their death or disability, and have therefore sanctioned interventions as being in the best interests of the child, in the face of the child's competent objection, eg transfusion in Jehovah's Witness patients, heart transplantation in cardiomyopathy. In contrast, parents may refuse treatment for their child when the burdens are likely to outweigh treatments, so that the offered treatment is arguably not in the child's best interests. It is inevitable that there will be situations in which children with identical conditions will receive very different treatments, depending on the wishes of the parents. This can be defended by the need to respect the autonomous choices of parents who will have to bear some of the burdens of the treatment or its outcome. This is especially likely to be the case with extremely premature infants, in whom the risk of significant mortality and morbidity is high, as illustrated by the findings of the EPICure studies and the recent publication from the Nuffield Council on Bioethics.

For a baby born alive at 23 weeks' gestation, parents may refuse treatment that they do not believe to be in their baby's best interests. However, matters are different for duodenal atresia in Down syndrome, in whom failure to operate will lead to the child's death. In the B case of 1981, the judge held that a child with Down syndrome should undergo surgery unless it were the case that the child's life would be so demonstrably awful that it would be unreasonable to expect him to bear it. Finally, courts are reluctant to impose the wishes of parents on children when the resultant burdens on the child will be great. In the case of the pregnant teenager who has been assessed as meeting the criteria of the Abortion Act and who is deemed to have the capacity to consent, the mother's refusal does not outweigh the child's consent. This is partly because it would be unethical to force a teenager to carry, deliver, and care for a baby that she did not want, and partly because of the harms that might accrue from overturning someone's competent consent.

7.8   Utilitarian moral theories: A C D E

Utilitarianism is a type of consequentialist moral theory in which the best consequences are those in which human happiness is maximised and harms are minimised for all relevant persons involved. An action is morally correct if it maximises welfare or individual preferences – 'the greatest good for the greatest number'. Some kind of formal calculation of risks/benefits is necessary and justifies reflective, evidence-based, audited practice. It involves making some assessment of reasonably foreseeable consequences, but doesn't require full precision. Application of a moral theory in which consequences do matter and in which there is an attempt to quantify benefits and burdens does provide individuals with an answer as to what action they should choose. However, other factors such as psychological disposition and emotional responses may interfere with the ability to perform a utilitarian calculus.

Children do not have special moral claims because they happen to be weak and vulnerable; whether they do or do not merit special treatment depends on the circumstances and the interests of others involved. Withdrawal of life-sustaining treatment from a sick infant can be justified because it minimises harms and suffering for the infant concerned. Although parents may object and suffer harms if their wishes are overridden, the interests of others also need to be considered. For example, staff on neonatal units may suffer harms if they are forced to provide treatment in which benefits are outweighed by burdens. Consequences for units in such circumstances could be difficulties in recruitment and retention of staff. Prolonging life-sustaining treatment may also mean that babies who might otherwise benefit from intensive care cannot be admitted to the unit. Application of the principle of utility is 'person-neutral' – no one counts as more than one – and hence it is democratic. Thus an action that benefits a large number – by conferring herd immunity, for example – is justified, even though a few may suffer severe consequences in terms of side-effects of immunisation.

7.9   Children's rights: B E

The United Nations (UN) Convention has been ratified by the UK Government, but it does not form part of UK law. UK Human Rights legislation is based on the European Human Rights declaration of the early 1950s. As such, it makes no specific provision for children, and the rights that it grants are mostly not absolute and they can be overridden in circumstances in which it is proportionate to do so. The UN Convention sets out in 42 articles a number of rights that children ought to enjoy. Its key principles include the following:

- Any decision or action concerning children as individuals or a group must have their best interests as a primary consideration.
- A child who is capable of forming his/her views has a right to express them freely.
- A child's view should be given due weight in accordance with that child's age and maturity.

Other UN Convention articles confirm the rights to freedom of expression (A13), the highest attainable standards of healthcare and rehabilitation from illness (A24), privacy (A16), freedom from discrimination (A2), and the right to family life and to hold religious beliefs. A child's right to life must be balanced against the obligation not to provide treatment that is inhuman and degrading and that confers more harms than benefits. Hence, there may be circumstances in which withdrawing life-sustaining treatment does not infringe a child's rights. In UKHRA terms, judgments involve balancing the above rights and obligations to determine what is in the best interests of the child. The fact that children have rights does not entail that they have to take the burden of decision-making if they do not want to do so. Under the age of 18 years in England and Wales, and under 16 years in Scotland, children can defer decisions to those who are legally entitled to make them on their behalf.

Best of Five Answers

7.10 E: Admit child to the ward, observe, and investigate further

The most likely explanation for the clinical presentation in a pre-ambulant baby is non-accidental injury, especially as there is evidence of a spiral fracture (which needs confirmation by formal radiological reporting). In these circumstances, it is important that a full assessment is carried out. This will include exclusion of clotting abnormality by appropriate studies and a skeletal survey to determine the presence of other fractures and to determine whether there is a generalised bony abnormality. There will also need to be a full social work assessment; realistically, that will not happen out of hours unless the child is at acute risk and the parents are not co-operative. It follows that option A is inappropriate because it precludes assessment and exposes the baby to further risk when non-accidental injury is already the most likely explanation. Equally, option B is also inappropriate, because abnormal clotting studies will not exclude the diagnosis of non-accidental injury and waiting for results in casualty leads to stress. The evidence base suggests that spiral fracture is a more reliable indicator of non-accidental injury. A skeletal survey is necessary, but in most cases these are not performed 'out of hours' or as outpatient procedures. They need to be performed by a skilled radiographer, and need to be interpreted by a radiologist with expertise in paediatrics. Finally, although a social work assessment is necessary, it is unlikely that this can be done rapidly, even by a member of the emergency team, and this provides extra tension, with the likely response that the mother will try to leave the department, having been frustrated with the wait and apprehensive of the involvement of social services.

The best option in these circumstances is to admit the baby for the purposes of carrying out the necessary assessments to determine how they came about their injuries. If there is refusal to co-operate, then a Police Protection Order can be sought.

7.11 D: Ask for a Court Order before giving the transfusion

This girl is anaemic, with a tachycardia and a gallop rhythm. The implication is that she is in heart failure due to her anaemia, which in turn is caused by her leukaemia. She therefore requires transfusion before her condition deteriorates further: transfusion is in her medical best interests. She clearly requires careful observation to determine how stable, or not, her condition is. If chemotherapy is given without transfusion, she is likely to become more anaemic, and will be placed at significant risk; this management will increase the urgency of her need for transfusion.

Although it is possible to argue that the family's religious beliefs are putting the girl at risk of significant harm, obtaining a Police Protection Order will not of itself enable a transfusion to be given, and may cause more alienation of the family by conflating child protection with clinical need. The urgency of the need for a blood transfusion depends upon the girl's clinical state. With the details given, transfusion is not immediately necessary to save her life or to prevent long-term harms, so it would be unwise to proceed against everyone's wishes unless there were agreement by an independent clinician that this was the case.

Although it is 1700 h, it is possible to obtain an urgent judicial ruling as to whether transfusion is in the girl's best interests. In reaching decisions, judges have visited sick children to ascertain for themselves the child's wishes and preferences, and to assess their competence in decision making. The involvement of an independent arbitration system also may help to defuse conflict, and provides both parents and child the opportunity to give their views. It is likely at present that courts will sanction life-sustaining treatment in these circumstances, but this may not always be the case, especially when refusal is persistently given by a young person who is felt to have the capacity to do so. It is helpful to know whether the girl is competent, and an appropriate professional to carry out this is a psychiatrist. However, as indicated, it is possible to overrule the wishes of a competent child if it is in their best interests to do so. If the girl is not competent, the persistent refusal of the family will still need legal review. Obtaining a psychiatric opinion is unlikely to obviate the need for legal review, and might cause further delay.

7.12 C: Arrange for Jim to have an assessment of his capacity to consent to treatment

Jim is at a developmental a stage when his testes are able to produce gametes (sperm). The provisions of the Human Fertilisation and Embryology Act 1990 apply here. Essentially, these currently require that those donating gametes should provide written consent. The consent of a proxy will not do, so that Jim's parents are unable to provide consent, even if they are able to do so with respect to Jim's treatment for his non-Hodgkin's lymphoma. Therefore it is important to assess Jim, to determine whether he is competent to consent. This has to be done in a sensitive manner and proceed at Jim's own pace, because he is unlikely to have thought about the issues involved. Moreover, there may be time pressures to commence treatment that reduce time available for discussion. Jim may not have masturbated, and may therefore have difficulties in producing a sample, which in any case may be of poor quality. If collection of sperm by masturbation is not possible, then other techniques that are less invasive than testicular biopsy can be used, and these may have less risk. It may be inappropriate to request sperm donation from those whose chances of survival are poor. It is possible that future assisted reproduction techniques will enable the use of any sperm that Jim will be able to produce when he becomes an adult, provided that he survives his non-Hodgkin's lymphoma. However, it is not possible to guarantee to the family that Jim will be fine. Although his parents can consent to the procedure to extract gametes, they cannot consent to their storage on Jim's behalf. Proposed amendments to the 1990 Act may alter this situation, with Jim and/or his parents able to give consent to storage. It is therefore important that up-to-date legal advice is sought.

7.13 B: From both parents

One consent is all that is required to protect a doctor from claims of negligence or from accusations of criminal common assault. The biological mother would be the most likely person to have parental responsibility for this child. Oral consent is perfectly adequate in law, but has the disadvantage that the existence of such consent may be hard to verify at a later date. This concern is increased when obtaining consent over the telephone, although it is still potentially valid. It can be difficult to be sure that the person giving consent is the one who actually has parental responsibility, even when meeting face to face. Over the telephone, there is more uncertainty. For this reason, both NHS Trusts and defence lawyers regard written consent as mandatory. For surgery performed on children for cosmetic, social or religious reasons, obtaining consent from both parents is encouraged and is considered to be best practice. A 12-year-old boy may certainly have sufficient capacity to give consent for this procedure, but it is likely that the surgery is being performed at his parents' request, so it would be marginally better to confirm their consent, rather than rely exclusively on his.

EMQ Answers

7.14 Consent

1. **G: Parent with parental responsibility**
2. **F: Biological father**

7.15 Capacity

1. **C: Person aged 18 years**
2. **A: Person with Gillick competence**

8. Gastroenterology and Nutrition

Multiple True–False Questions

8.1 Hydrolysed formulas include:

- [ ] A Pepti-Junior
- [ ] B Neocate
- [ ] C Infatrini
- [ ] D Enfamil AR
- [ ] E Elemental-028

8.2 The Department of Health recommends

- [ ] A exclusive breast-feeding of healthy infants for the first 6 months of life
- [ ] B vitamin A and D supplementation for formula-fed infants older than 6 months taking < 500 mL formula/day
- [ ] C goat's milk as a suitable substitute for cow's milk
- [ ] D introduction of solids from 17 weeks of age
- [ ] E vitamin A and D supplementation for all children up to 5 years of age

8.3 Diarrhoea

- [ ] A is seen in appendicitis
- [ ] B is a recognised feature of toxic shock syndrome
- [ ] C may be bloody in toddler's diarrhoea
- [ ] D is associated with phototherapy
- [ ] E may be absent at first presentation of Crohn's disease

8.4 Consequences of re-feeding syndrome include:

- [ ] A hypokalaemia
- [ ] B hyperphosphataemia
- [ ] C hypomagnesaemia
- [ ] D tetany
- [ ] E cardiac dysrhythmias

8.5   Oral rehydration solution

☐ A   contains 90 mmol/L sodium in the Western world
☐ B   contains a base such as citrate
☐ C   should be given instead of breast milk in acute gastroenteritis
☐ D   should be given for the first 24 hours of a diarrhoeal illness
☐ E   is recommended for protracted diarrhoeal illnesses

8.6   Hirschprung's disease

☐ A   is associated with a gene on chromosome 10
☐ B   is associated with central hypoventilation syndrome
☐ C   is associated with a decrease in acylcholinesterase-positive nerve fibres in the lamina propria
☐ D   has an incidence of 1 in 5000
☐ E   is familial in short-segment disease

Best of Five Questions

8.7   Blood is found in the stool of an otherwise healthy, breast-fed term infant at 3 days. What is the MOST useful investigation?

☐ A   Clotting studies
☐ B   Apt's test
☐ C   pH probe study
☐ D   Radioallergosorbent test (RAST) to cow's milk protein
☐ E   Skin-prick test to cow's milk protein

8.8   On annual screening bloods, an 8-year-old child with type 1 diabetes mellitus who has no gastrointestinal symptoms has the following results:

IgA   2.2 g/L   (normal range 0.7–2.5 g/L)
Tissue transglutaminase IgA   30 U/mL (normal range 0–4 U/mL)

Which of the following is the MOST appropriate action?

☐ A   Commence gluten-free diet
☐ B   Repeat coeliac serology in 1 year and continue current diet
☐ C   Repeat coeliac serology if gastrointestinal symptoms develop
☐ D   Refer for small-bowel biopsy
☐ E   Perform small-bowel biopsy if gastrointestinal symptoms develop

8.9 **A 15-year-old Eastern European refugee presents with a 2-month history of right iliac fossa pain, weight loss, amenorrhoea, and a 1-month history of diarrhoea. Investigations show:**

Haemoglobin	9.1 g/dL
White blood cells	11.2×10^9/L
Neutrophils	8.2×10^9/L
Platelets	719×10^9/L
Mean cell volume	68 fL
Albumin	29 g/L

What is the MOST likely diagnosis?

☐ A   Laxative abuse
☐ B   Tuberculosis
☐ C   Appendix abscess
☐ D   Pelvic inflammatory disease
☐ E   Crohn's disease

8.10 **In a child with suspected gastro-oesophageal reflux, which of the following is the MOST useful investigation?**

☐ A   Barium meal
☐ B   Barium swallow
☐ C   pH study
☐ D   Oesophageal biopsy
☐ E   Radionucleotide milk scan

8.11 **In a child in whom pancreatic insufficiency is suspected and cystic fibrosis has been excluded, the MOST useful investigation would be which of the following?**

☐ A   Stool α_1-antitrypsin
☐ B   Stool chromatography
☐ C   Stool faecal calprotectin
☐ D   Stool faecal elastase
☐ E   Stool microscopy for faecal fats

8.12 A girl aged 2 years presents with generalised fatigue. Basic investigations show a borderline low haemoglobin, low serum iron, and increased transferrin. MCV (mean cell volume) is 76 fL. She has a mild thrombocytosis. Coeliac screen is negative. Of the five options below, which is the MOST likely cause?

- ☐ A Dietary
- ☐ B Occult blood loss
- ☐ C Gastro-oesophageal reflux
- ☐ D Infection
- ☐ E Haemoglobinopathy

8.13 In a child referred with suspected peanut allergy, what would the next best step be?

- ☐ A Peanut challenge
- ☐ B Advice and dietetic input with regard to peanut exclusion
- ☐ C Skin-prick test
- ☐ D Supply of an adrenaline (epinephrine) pen
- ☐ E IgE radioallergosorbent (RAST) testing

Extended Matching Questions

8.14 Theme: Vomiting

A   Hirschprung's disease
B   Necrotising enterocolitis
C   Galactosaemia
D   Urinary tract infection
E   Intussusception
F   Pyloric stenosis
G   Gastro-oesophageal reflux
H   Gastroenteritis
I   Overfeeding
J   Cystic fibrosis

For each of the following scenarios, select the most likely diagnosis from the above list of possible diagnoses. Each option may be used once, more than once, or not at all.

☐   1. A 5-week-old breast-fed baby boy presents with a 2-week history of progressively worsening non-bilious vomiting after feeds. He is thriving.

☐   2. A 10-month-old baby presents with a 2-day history of fever, diarrhoea and vomiting. He has associated episodes of irritability and pallor, associated with drawing up of his legs.

☐   3. A 5-day-old baby born at term presents with a serum bilirubin of 558 μmol/L, blood sugar of 1.9 mmol/L, and a positive blood culture for Gram-negative rods.

8.15 Theme: Abdominal pain

A   Ulcerative colitis
B   Crohn's disease
C   Cystic fibrosis
D   Coeliac disease
E   Gastro-oesophageal reflux
F   Wilms' tumour
G   Hirschsprung's disease
H   Constipation
I   Abdominal migraine
J   Diabetes

For each of the following scenarios, select the most likely diagnosis from the above list of possible diagnoses. Each option may be used once, more than once, or not at all.

☐ 1. An 11-year-old girl presents with recurrent abdominal pain over 3 months. She is well in herself and has recently started at secondary school. There is no history of weight loss. She is out of school more than half of the time. She was previously well, and there is no relevant family history. Tissue transglutaminase is positive.

☐ 2. A 14-year-old girl presents with a 6-week history of abdominal pain, bloody diarrhoea and weight loss. Platelet count is increased, but other inflammatory markers are normal. Stool culture is negative.

☐ 3. A 13-year-old boy presents with a 6-month history of recurrent abdominal pain. The pain occurs mostly in the evenings, just before he goes to sleep. He is not missing school. There is a past history of recurrent abdominal pain, although the last time it was a major problem was when he was 11 years old. There is an abdominal mass. Basic bloods are normal.

MT–F Answers

8.1 Hydrolysed formulas: A B E

A hydrolysed formula is one in which the protein is broken down into oligopeptides and peptides. In elemental formulas, the protein is further broken down into single amino acids. Neocate and Elemental-O28 are hydrolysed formulas that are elemental. If a cow's milk protein intolerance or allergy is suspected, an extensively hydrolysed formula such as Pepti-Junior or an amino acid formula such as Neocate should be given.

- Pepti-junior: 67 kcal/100 mL, 50% medium-chain triglycerides (MCT); has the lowest osmolality (190 mosmol/kg water); good if diarrhoea is a problem.
- Neocate (suitable from birth): 71 kcal/100 mL, 5% MCT. Osmolality 360 mosmol/kg water.
- Elemental-028 (suitable for infants older than 1 year): 100 kcal/100 mL; has a high osmolality (496 mosmol/kg water).

Other hydrolysed formulas include: Prejomin, Nutramigen and Flexical. Infatrini is a high-energy formula (100 kcal/100 mL), and Enfamil AR is a reflux formula that contains rice starch and has a normal consistency in the bottle but thickens on contact with gastric acid. Indications for the use of hydrolysed formulas include:

- cow's milk protein intolerance
- enteropathies (post-gastroenteritis)
- post necrotising enterocolitis
- short gut
- severe eczema
- Crohn's disease.

In infants in whom there is a strong family history of atopy and breast-feeding is not possible, a hydrolysed formula can be considered, as there is some evidence this will reduce the risk of the atopy in the infant. Breast-feeding remains the best strategy to reduce subsequent allergies. In these infants particularly, weaning should be discouraged before 17 weeks, and those foods regarded as allergenic (eg eggs, cow's milk, soya, wheat and fish) should not be introduced into the diet until the infant is 6 months of age.

8.2 Department of Health recommendations: A B E

Recommendations by the Department of Health include a daily dose of vitamins A, C, and D for:

- breast-fed infants from 6 months (or 1 month if there is any doubt about the mother's vitamin status during pregnancy)
- formula-fed infants older than 6 months who are fed less than 500 mL infant formula per day
- children under 5 years.

Vitamin D supplementation is especially important for children with dark skin (Asian, African, Afro-Caribbean and Middle-Eastern), those living in northern areas of the UK and children who are selective eaters. Exposure to sunlight is the major source of vitamin D as few foods naturally contain high levels of vitamin D. People with dark skin require more time in the sun to make vitamin D compared with white people. The incidence of rickets is rising in the UK and the USA. The role of Vitamin D in rickets is well established but this vitamin could have important protective roles in other diseases such as cancer, diabetes and heart disease. A new scheme called 'Healthy Start' replaces the Welfare Food Scheme and provides **free** 'Healthy Start vitamin supplements' from 6 months until the 4th birthday for infants whose parents are receiving Income Support and other means of financial support.

For women, the Department of Health recommends:

- 10 μg of vitamin D each day for pregnant women and those who are breast-feeding
- 400 μg of folic acid for those who may become pregnant up to the 12th week of pregnancy.

From March 2007, infant milks based on goat's milk protein will no longer be sold in the UK. Goat's milk preparations are not a suitable source of nutrition for infants (under 1 year of age). The protein in goat's milk is very similar to that in cow's milk, so it is not an appropriate substitute milk in cow's milk allergy, as there is a potential for cross-reactivity. It is also unsuitable for babies with lactose intolerance, as it contains levels of lactose similar to those in cow's milk formulas. Six months is the recommended age for the introduction of solid foods for infants, whether breast- or formula-fed. Introduction of solids before 17 weeks is not advised.

8.3   Diarrhoea: A B D E

Diarrhoea is seen in appendicitis. An initial diagnosis of gastroenteritis is often made in patients with diarrhoea, which can delay treatment of an appendicitis. Diarrhoea can be marked in post-ileal or retrocaecal appendicitis.

Toxic shock syndrome is a serious but uncommon medical emergency caused by an exotoxin-producing strain of *Staphylococcus aureus*; 50% are tampon-related (toxic shock syndrome toxin 1 [TSST-1]) and 50% are caused by initially trivial wounds, burns or surgical incisions that develop a localised infection (TSST-1 or staphylococcal enterotoxin B [SEB] or C [SEC]). (Note that, strictly, toxic shock syndrome [TSS] differs from streptococcal toxic shock syndrome [STSS] caused by streptococcal pyogenic exotoxin A [SPEA] — often a result of deep-seated infections such as fasciitis and myositis.) Symptoms of TSS include:

- sudden high fever > 38.8 °C
- vomiting
- profuse watery diarrhoea
- confluent sunburn-like rash (red and flat)
- fainting/dizziness
- myalgia
- confusion
- desquamation of the palms and soles 1–2 weeks after onset of illness
- conjunctivitis.

TSS can rapidly progress to severe, intractable hypotension and multi-organ failure. Emergency treatment includes resuscitation (ABC), oxygen, restoration of blood pressure, intravenous antibiotics (eg clindamycin) and intravenous immunoglobulins (including removal of the source, eg tampon).

Only 25% of Crohn's disease presents with the triad of abdominal pain, weight loss and diarrhoea. The majority (approximately 75%) will complain of abdominal pain. Many present in a non-classic manner, with vague symptoms such as lethargy or anorexia with mild abdominal discomfort. Extra-intestinal manifestations may dominate the clinical presentation in children, causing delay in diagnosis.

Toddler's diarrhoea is the most common cause of persistent loose stools in pre-school children. It **never** causes blood in the stools, by definition. It is often referred to as 'peas and carrots syndrome' due to the presence of undigested vegetables in the stool. The child is otherwise well and thriving, and has normal stool microscopy and reducing sugars. An inappropriate 'healthy adult-style diet' may be contributing. The following advice should be given:

- Avoid low-fat diets. Toddlers should have a diet with 35–45% fat.
- Limit intake of squash and fruit juices.
- Avoid high-fibre diets.

8.4   Re-feeding syndrome: A C D E

Re-feeding syndrome was first described in Japanese prisoners after World War II. It is a potentially fatal consequence of severe fluid and electrolyte shifts and their associated complications in malnourished patients undergoing re-feeding. Typically, it is seen in the first 4 days of re-feeding, whether parenteral or enteral. Consequences of re-feeding syndrome include:

- Hyperinsulinism: due to the sudden shift from fat metabolism (in the undernourished) to primarily carbohydrate metabolism.
- Depleted electrolyte pool: hyperinsulinism causes an intracellular shift of glucose along with phosphate, magnesium and potassium.
- Increase demand for phosphorylated intermediates such as ATP, due to the shift from fat metabolism (which does not require phosphorylated intermediates) to glucose metabolism.
- Deficiency of micronutrients: the glucose load increases the metabolic demand for thiamine.

Ideally, it is necessary to be aware of 'at risk' patients (poor intake, malnourished) and to check plasma biochemistry before and during re-feeding and slowly increase calorie delivery. General principles of management include:

- replacement of phosphate, potassium and magnesium
- consider thiamine replacement
- consider need for other vitamins
- increase feeds slowly.

Consequences of low phosphate, potassium and magnesium can be:

cardiac:	arrhythmia, cardiac arrest, congestive cardiac failure
respiratory:	respiratory depression
neuromuscular:	confusion, coma, rhabdomyolysis
renal:	polyuria, polydipsia
metabolic:	tetany (caused by low magnesium)
hepatic:	encephalopathy
gastrointestinal:	constipation and diarrhoea

8.5   Oral rehydration solution: B

Between 1980 and 2000, the use of oral rehydration solution decreased the number of children under 5 years of age dying of diarrhoea from 4.6 million to 1.8 million – a reduction of 60%. The World Health Organisation (WHO) recommends 90 mmol/L sodium, which is specifically designed for cholera. Oral rehydration solution for use in developed countries has a lower sodium (45–50 mmol/L), typically 35–60 mmol/L in European preparations. Home-made preparations usually contain an excess of salt, putting children at risk of hypernatraemic dehydration. Parents should also be warned of the dangers of giving sugar-free drinks (as the only source of fluid and calories) to their children during diarrhoeal illnesses. In the case of children with acute gastroenteritis:

- Breast-fed infants should continue to breast-feed along with oral rehydration solution, to correct dehydration and replace stool losses.
- Formula-fed infants should be given suitable oral rehydration solution for 3–4 hours, followed by rapid introduction of normal feeding.
- Following gastroenteritis, carbohydrate intolerance may be seen (especially after rotavirus) as a result of brush-border destruction. If reducing substances in the stool are positive (> 0.5%), a lactose-free diet (for approximately 6 weeks) is recommended.
- Protracted diarrhoeal illnesses require specialist assessment, and immunodeficiency states such as acquired immune deficiency syndrome (AIDS) should always be considered.

The most common causes of loose stools are gastrointestinal infections or food poisoning. The presence of blood in loose stools suggests *Campylobacter*, *Shigella*, or *Salmonella*, but one should always consider

Cause	Organism	Source / comment
Unknown		In up to 50% of cases in developing and developed countries, the cause may not be identified
Viral	Rotavirus (most common) Adenovirus Small round viruses Astroviruses	
Bacterial	Bloody diarrhoea (all notifiable diseases) *Campylobacter*	Undercooked meat, especially poultry; unpasteurised milk, and untreated water
	Shigella spp.	*S. dysenteriae* form may cause haemolytic uraemic syndrome
	Salmonella spp. Enteropathic *Escherichia coli* Enterotoxic *E. coli* O157:H7 Non-bloody diarrhoea *Vibrio cholerae* *Yersinia enterocolitis*	Meat, raw eggs, dairy Associated with haemolytic uraemic syndrome Raw pork and pork products
Protozoal	*Cryptosporidium* spp. *Giardia* spp. *Entamoeba histolytica*	Especially immunocompromised host Water-borne Amoebic dysentery

intussusception, ulcerative colitis and haemolytic uraemic syndrome as part of the differential diagnosis.

The differential diagnosis is:

- other infections: ENT (otitis media, tonsillitis), pneumonia, septicaemia, urinary tract infections
- intussusception
- haemolytic uraemic syndrome
- pyloric stenosis
- acute appendicitis.

8.6 Hirschprung's disease: A B D

Hirschprung's disease is associated with the *RET* proto-oncogene on chromosome 10, Down syndrome (2–15%), central hypoventilation, and other congenital anomalies. It has an incidence of 1 in 5000. More males are affected than females, except in long-segment disease (4–7%), which is familial, with equal sex incidence. Ultra-short-segment Hirschprung's disease is very rare, and can present significant diagnostic difficulty. Diagnosis of Hirschprung's disease is based on rectal biopsy. Histology shows an **excess** of acylcholinesterase activity. There is an absence of ganglion cells in the myenteric plexus of the most distal large bowel. Patients usually present with delayed passage of meconium (> 24 hours). Most children with Hirschprung's disease have never had a normal bowel habit. In the case of total colonic / small bowel involvement the prognosis is poor. Bowel obstruction may be relieved by explosive decompression following rectal examination. Surgery is usually with excision of the affected portion, with delayed pull-through, when the infant is aged around 6 months. Enterocolitis can occur before or after surgery, and is associated with *Clostridium difficile* enterotoxin. The enterocolitis can result in severe systemic collapse requiring resuscitation, broad-spectrum antibiotics and emergency defunctioning colostomy.

Best of Five Answers

8.7 B: Apt's test

This is more useful than clotting studies to determine the origin of the bleed. When a newborn vomits or passes blood per rectum, it is essential to determine whether the blood originates from the mother or the baby. Apt's test differentiates fetal blood from maternal blood in the evaluation of bloody stools. Maternal blood can be swallowed at delivery from the birth canal or from cracked nipples during breast-feeding. Maternal blood is

made up of adult haemoglobin, which has two α and two β subunits. Fetal haemoglobin has two α and two γ subunits which are resistant to alkali denaturation. When mixed with sodium hydrochloride:
fetal Hb … remains pink
adult Hb … will turn yellow/brown.
There are several causes of rectal bleeding in term neonates:

- swallowed maternal blood
- haemorrhagic disease of the newborn, an important cause that requires prompt treatment
- cow's milk enterocolitis
- necrotising enterocolitis; much more common in pre-term neonates
- volvulus
- Hirschprung's enterocolitis
- use of non-steroidal anti-inflammatory drugs (NSAIDs) such as indometacin (eg for closure of a patent duct)
- maternal use of drugs such as aspirin or phenobarbital in late pregnancy.

Haemorrhagic disease of the newborn can be early or late in onset. The early form (day 2–6 of life) is caused by vitamin K deficiency and subsequent deficiency of factors II, VII, IX and X. It usually presents with gastrointestinal haemorrhage, umbilical stump bleeding, nose bleeds, or intracranial haemorrhage. The late-onset form (8 days to 6 months) is more commonly characterised by intracranial haemorrhage. High-risk patients include those who have not received prophylactic vitamin K, either by intramuscular or adequate oral dose, infants who are pre-term, small for gestational age, breast-fed, and whose mothers have received anticonvulsant therapy (phenytoin, phenobarbital). Prothrombin time (PT) and activated partial thromboplastin time (APTT) are prolonged. Treatment is with fresh frozen plasma and intravenous vitamin K, with or without blood transfusion. There is no proved association between intramuscular vitamin K and childhood cancer. The current recommendation is to give all babies either a single intramuscular dose or three doses of oral vitamin K (at birth, 1–2 weeks, and 6 weeks) to prevent the condition.

8.8   D: Refer for small-bowel biopsy

Most endocrinologists and gastroenterologists would refer this patient for endoscopy, but there is some debate as to the exact timing of this referral. For the given question, referral for small-bowel biopsy is the most appropriate answer. The prevalence of coeliac disease in type 1 diabetes is about 4%. Management is by gluten exclusion. Positive serology should revert to negative over time. If there is no decline in antibody levels after

6 months, adherence to the diet should be reviewed. The serology is suggestive, and diagnosis is confirmed by small-bowel biopsy demonstrating abnormal duodenal mucosa:

- partial or complete villous atrophy
- crypt hyperplasia
- increased intra-epithelial lymphocytes in the lamina propria

in the presence of positive serology on a gluten-containing diet. It is crucial that gluten intake is adequate at the time of the biopsy. In general, a minimum of 10 g gluten should be eaten on a daily basis (equivalent to two slices of white bread). This is best confirmed by dietetic assessment.

There should be complete resolution of symptoms on a strict gluten-free diet. Children who were supposedly asymptomatic may, in retrospect, have had a mild impairment of growth, along with symptoms of irritability, lethargy and abdominal distension before adopting a gluten-free diet. The risks of non-treatment in symptomatic patients include impaired growth and pubertal development, increased risk of osteoporosis, infertility, and gastrointestinal malignancy. The assumption is that asymptomatic children will have the same long-term benefits of a gluten-free diet, and that all biopsy-positive children should be treated. Currently, there is no evidence to demonstrate improvement in short-term diabetic control on a gluten-free diet. Medium- and long-term effects are still unknown. It is unclear whether treating coeliac disease has an effect on the subsequent development of other autoimmune diseases in this group of patients.

In individuals with selective IgA deficiency, IgA from other individuals (eg blood products received via transfusions) may be recognised as a foreign protein and result in the production of anti-IgA antibodies in the recipient. Thus patients with selective IgA deficiency (associated with coeliac disease) should receive a card (much like a steroid-risk card) warning of potential anaphylaxis and adverse reactions to blood transfusions and blood products.

8.9 E: Crohn's disease

The three main differential diagnoses are Crohn's disease, appendix abscess and tuberculosis (TB). Crohn's disease can explain all the symptoms, including the iron-deficiency anaemia. It is the most likely diagnosis. In Crohn's disease, inflammatory markers (erythrocyte sedimentation rate [ESR] and C-reactive protein [CRP]) and platelets are characteristically increased, along with evidence of anaemia and hypoalbuminaemia. In children, Crohn's disease is more common than ulcerative colitis, and the above parameters are more likely to be abnormal. The amenorrhoea suggests that the problem is chronic. Growth failure and delayed sexual development are common. Crohn's disease is a chronic inflammatory disorder involving the gastrointestinal tract from the mouth to the anus. For this reason, upper (gastroscopy) and lower (ileo-colonoscopy) gastrointestinal endoscopies are used to provide a histological diagnosis following barium radiology. Radiological examination can sometimes better define the disease extent and presence of complications, such as small-bowel strictures and fistulae. The aims of treatment in Crohn's disease are to induce disease remission and facilitate normal growth and development. These are achieved through the use of:

- **Enteral nutrition**. Whole-protein (polymeric) nutrition given as **sole** therapy for 6–8 weeks will induce remission in 60–80% of patients, depending on case selection. Crohn's disease with **ileal** involvement tends to respond well. Between 110% and 120% of the recommended nutritional requirement is usually required. Food is slowly re-introduced over 2–4 weeks at the end of the treatment course. Multidisciplinary management is essential.
- **Corticosteroids**. These are effective at inducing remission – either orally or intravenously in the case of severe pancolitis. Supplements of calcium and vitamin D should be considered during steroid therapy.
- **5-Aminosalicylates**. Mesalazine has fewer side-effects than sulfasalazine.
- **Azathioprine**. This is a highly effective maintenance agent for moderate to severe Crohn's disease, and is indicated in frequently relapsing disease and in those with steroid toxicity. Side-effects include bone marrow suppression and pancreatitis. Regular monitoring of the full blood count and amylase is required.
- **Antibiotics**. These should be broad-spectrum if disease is fulminant. Oral metronidazole may help peri-anal disease.
- **Second-line immunosuppression**. Methotrexate, ciclosporin, and anti-TNF monoclonal antibodies (infliximab) may be considered for cases unresponsive to the above therapies.
- **Surgery**. Indicated for localised disease (eg strictures), abscess, or disease resistant to medical therapy.

Differentiating Crohn's disease from TB is important, as steroid treatment can be detrimental in undiagnosed TB. Biopsy is indicated, but computed tomography and imaging may be very informative. In endemic areas, a trial of empirical TB treatment might be given. The incidence of TB is increasing in the UK, particularly among immigrants (traditionally considered to be from Africa and Asia) and those with human immunodeficiency virus (HIV). The prevalence of TB amongst Eastern European countries is higher than in the UK. Clinical features of intestinal TB include weight loss, anaemia, night sweats and abdominal pain. Malabsorption, obstruction and haemorrhage may occur. Perforation is less frequent than in Crohn's disease. Right iliac fossa pain or mass may be present, as ileo-caecal involvement is seen in 80% patients with gastrointestinal TB (probably because of the abundance of lymphoid tissue – Peyer's patches).

A diagnosis of appendix abscess should be considered in any child who has initial symptoms of appendicitis that settle and recur with chronic gastrointestinal symptoms and raised inflammatory markers. In the case described, the raised inflammatory markers go against a diagnosis of laxative abuse. Performing pregnancy tests and screening for sexually transmitted disease, including pelvic inflammatory disease, should be considered in all teenagers presenting with abdominal pain.

8.10 C: pH study

Although many children with reflux do not need further investigation, if performed, a pH study is the most useful; it is the gold-standard test for acid reflux, although alkaline reflux will be missed. The strength of the investigation is that it can be done over a 24-hour period and it relates temporally with events (feeds, apnoea). Barium radiology is not particularly sensitive or specific, but will pick up anatomical problems such as malrotation or stricture. A nuclear medicine 'milk' scan will assess acid or alkali reflux following a physiological meal. Upper gastrointestinal endoscopy with biopsy will detect oesophagitis, but can be negative in the presence of reflux.

8.11 D: Stool faecal elastase

Elastase is a pancreas-specific enzyme that is stable during intestinal transport and is stable in faeces. It is a reliable, indirect marker of pancreatic function, although false positives can occur in short gut and bacterial overgrowth. Alpha$_1$-antitrypsin is a serum protein; it is not present in the diet. It has the same molecular weight as albumin. Faecal levels reflect enteric protein loss (protein-losing enteropathy). Stool chromatography will detect malabsorbed carbohydrate. Calprotectin is a neutrophil protein, stable in faeces, and is found in both adults and children to be a simple and non-invasive measure of bowel inflammation.

8.12 A: Dietary

The most common cause of iron-deficiency anaemia is dietary, involving particularly prolonged or excessive milk feeding. Other causes include chronic blood loss (eg oesophagitis) and malabsorption. Dietary sources of iron include cereals, red meat (particularly liver), fresh fruit and green vegetables. Iron is absorbed from the proximal small bowel. Vitamin C, gastric acid and protein improve absorption. Deficiency causes hypochromic microcytic anaemia, associated with poor appetite and reduced intellectual function. A child with a haemoglobinopathy and iron deficiency would be expected to have a lower mean cell volume (MCV).

8.13 C: Skin-prick test

Peanut and nut allergy are being seen with increasing frequency. It is important to remember that peanuts are a vegetable rather than a true nut. Around 60–80% of children with peanut allergy are also allergic to other nuts. Reactions vary from mild urticaria to life-threatening anaphylaxis. First-line investigation involves skin-prick testing, which is useful, having high sensitivity and specificity. It is important to get the diagnosis right; many children have non-specific reactions during childhood and are labelled as peanut-allergic. Peanut avoidance is difficult and dietetic support is essential. Even when food labels do not list nuts among the ingredients, contamination might have occurred in trace amounts because of cross-contamination from other food production lines. There is some controversy as to whether all nuts should be avoided in peanut-allergic patients, and whether peanut oils can be given. The natural history suggests that children with early-onset allergy may grow out of it, although symptomatic reactions are more likely to persist if they occur in older children. Active management involves challenge of children whose skin-prick tests were negative for peanuts. This is clearly not without risk, and needs to be done in an inpatient setting with facilities for resuscitation.

EMQ Answers

8.14 Vomiting

1.   G: Gastro-oesophageal reflux

The main differentials are overfeeding and pyloric stenosis. However, the key points are that this child is breast-fed and less likely to be overfed, and that the child is thriving (not likely in pyloric stenosis). Gastro-oesphageal reflux is common, and a normal physiological phenomenon. Most cases improve with time as a result of adopting a more upright posture and intake of solids, but review of positioning and frequency and volume of feeds may be helpful. Indications for investigation and treatment include: faltering growth, refusal to feed or crying associated with feeding, or choking and apnoea after feeds. The gold standard for diagnosis of acid reflux is a pH probe, and reflux can be classified according to the percentage of time when the pH is < 4:

5–10%   mild
10–20% moderate
20–30% severe

Gastro-oesphageal reflux can be managed with thickeners (eg Gaviscon, Carobel). Specific treatments include:

- acid suppression (H_2-blockers, eg ranitidine)
- proton pump inhibitors (eg omeprazole)
- prokinetic drugs (eg domperidone, metoclopramide).

Note that cisapride is no longer licensed for use in children because of its association with prolonged QT syndrome. Surgery (fundoplication) is considered for reflux resistant to medical management.

2. E: Intussusception

The differentials include gastroenteritis and urinary tract infection, but **pallor** is key in combination with the other features, making intussusception the most likely diagnosis. Vomiting is an early feature and rapidly becomes bile-stained. Severe pain is a very common and important symptom. The characteristic stools are described as 'redcurrant jelly-like', but this is a relatively late sign. The classic triad of symptoms (not seen in all patients) is:

- abdominal pain (and drawing up of legs)
- bleeding per rectum
- palpable mass.

Peak incidence of intussusception occurs at age 6–9 months; more common in boys. The intussusception is usually ileo-caecal. A Meckel's diverticulum, polyp, Henoch–Schönlein purpura and lymphosarcoma are sometimes identified as causes, as they act as a 'lead point' for the intussusception. Ultrasound and plain abdominal radiography can confirm diagnosis. Careful attention to resuscitation is necessary – fluid boluses of up to 40 mL/kg may be necessary. With a short history, air-enema reduction may be attempted (contraindicated with signs of perforation); otherwise laparotomy is indicated. Recurrence of intussusception occurs in about 7% of patients and is more likely after enema reduction and within 2–3 days.

3. C: Galactosaemia

Although a rare autosomal recessive disorder, galactosaemia should be considered in all cases of severe early-onset jaundice and in neonates with *Escherichia coli* sepsis (Gram-negative rod). *E. coli* sepsis is seen in 25–50% of cases. Despite early treatment, there is usually developmental delay (particularly speech and feeding problems). Most affected women are infertile. The most common, type I or classical, galactosaemia is caused by galactose-1-phosphate uridyl transferase (Gal-1-PUT) deficiency. (Type II, galactokinase deficiency, results in cataracts only.) Babies may present with vomiting, diarrhoea, lethargy, poor feeding, hypoglycaemia, and a mixed jaundice. There may be later presentation with faltering growth, proximal tubulopathy (Fanconi syndrome) and rickets. Clotting is nearly always slightly prolonged, even in the absence of obvious major liver involvement. Note that jaundice, hepatomegaly and cataracts, seen in galactosaemia, may also be seen in congenital rubella. Diagnosis of galactosaemia depends on:

- presence of reducing substances in **urine** (Clinitest +ve; Clinistix for glucose –ve)
- levels of Gal-1-PUT in red blood cells
- (screening of the parents or carrier activity if the child has already received a transfusion).

There is rapid progression to irreversible severe learning difficulties, particularly involving speech, and cirrhosis in undiagnosed patients. In those diagnosed, management involves a strict lactose- / galactose-free diet for life. Milk is replaced with soya-based formula.

8.15 Abdominal Pain

1. D: Coeliac disease
The tissue transglutaminase antibody is highly sensitive and specific for coeliac disease. Coeliac serology should be investigated in any child with chronic gastrointestinal symptoms.

2. A: Ulcerative colitis
This could be either Crohn's disease or ulcerative colitis, but inflammatory markers are almost universally raised in Crohn's disease, and so the normal C-reactive protein (CRP) here favours ulcerative colitis.

3. H: Constipation
The presence of a mass, particularly if it will indent on palpation in a child with recurrent abdominal pain, is a pointer to chronic constipation, with faecal loading as a potential cause. This is a common cause of an abdominal mass. Obviously, in such a child there would need to be a low threshold for further investigation, including basic blood analyses with or without plain abdominal X-ray and ultrasound.

9. Genetics

Multiple True–False Questions

9.1 Prader–Willi syndrome

- [ ] A causes neonatal hypotonia
- [ ] B is associated with severe learning disability
- [ ] C is a common diagnosis in an obese child
- [ ] D does not affect fertility
- [ ] E is associated with diabetes and heart disease in early adult life

9.2 The following is true of congenital adrenal hyperplasia:

- [ ] A more girls than boys are diagnosed
- [ ] B there is an antenatal treatment to reduce virilisation
- [ ] C it is tested for in the neonatal screening programme
- [ ] D treatment can usually cease after puberty
- [ ] E carrier screening is not usually available for members of the wider family

9.3 In achondroplasia, features present in the majority of affected individuals include:

- [ ] A mesomelic shortening
- [ ] B hydrocephalus
- [ ] C Madelung deformity
- [ ] D trident hand
- [ ] E pronounced lumbar lordosis

9.4 The following is true of a child with neurofibromatosis type 1:

- [ ] A the child is likely to be infertile
- [ ] B there will be learning difficulties
- [ ] C if no neurofibromas have grown by the age of 10 years, it is unlikely that any will appear
- [ ] D Lisch nodules can affect vision
- [ ] E the diagnosis should be confirmed by mutation analysis of the *NF1* gene

9.5 Karyotyping is indicated in a patient with

☐ A suspected Down syndrome
☐ B unexplained developmental delay
☐ C galactosaemia
☐ D Treacher Collins syndrome
☐ E congenital adrenal hyperplasia

9.6 A couple are first cousins. The following is true:

☐ A their risk of having a baby with an autosomal recessive disorder is
       1 in 4
☐ B they should not have children
☐ C they have an increased risk of having a baby with ill-health in the
       first year
☐ D they are most likely to have healthy children
☐ E if there is a known recessive disorder in other family members, they
       should be offered testing

Best of Five Questions

**9.7 A pregnant woman tells you that she had a brother who died of
spinal muscular atrophy, and that her partner's sister's son has
recently been diagnosed with the condition, She wants to know
her risk of having an affected child. Which is the CLOSEST answer
from the list below?**

☐ A 6%
☐ B 25%
☐ C 25% if the fetus is male
☐ D 12.5%
☐ E 8%

**9.8 A baby has neonatal seizures. Which of the following is LEAST
likely to be the underlying diagnosis?**

☐ A Galactosaemia
☐ B Angelman syndrome
☐ C Rett syndrome in a male
☐ D Birth asphyxia
☐ E Arginosuccinicaciduria

9.9 A 35-year-old man is diagnosed with hereditary motor and sensory neuropathy (Charcot–Marie–Tooth [CMT] syndrome) on nerve conduction studies, having suffered weakness for many years. He wishes to have his 3-year-old son tested for the condition. The MOST appropriate first course of action is which of the following?

- ☐ A Collect DNA from the son for screening for a duplication in the *PMP22* gene, which causes CMT1
- ☐ B Arrange for nerve conduction studies on the child
- ☐ C Perform a neurological examination on the child
- ☐ D Collect DNA from the father for testing
- ☐ E Check the child's paternity

9.10 In a child with bilateral lens dislocation, mild joint limitation, and learning disability, the MOST likely diagnosis is which of the following?

- ☐ A Stickler syndrome
- ☐ B Marfan syndrome
- ☐ C Ehlers–Danlos syndrome
- ☐ D Homocystinuria
- ☐ E Benign familial joint hypermobility

9.11 A Turkish couple are concerned about their offspring risks, given that they are first cousins, although they have no family history of any genetic disorder. Which of the following would be the MOST appropriate testing to offer them?

- ☐ A Carrier testing for cystic fibrosis
- ☐ B Carrier testing for familial Mediterranean fever
- ☐ C Carrier testing for Gaucher's disease
- ☐ D Karyotyping on blood
- ☐ E Carrier testing for haemoglobinopathies

9.12 A 22-year-old woman who is pregnant tells you she had a sister who died as a baby from a severe atrioventricular septal defect associated with Down syndrome. She has no further information, but is concerned about her own risk of having a baby with Down syndrome. The MOST appropriate course of action is which one of the following?

☐ A Check her chromosomes, and proceed with routine maternal serum screening and anomaly scanning if they are normal

☐ B Check her chromosomes, and proceed with routine maternal serum screening and anomaly scanning if they show she carries a Robertsonian translocation between chromosomes 14 and 21

☐ C Offer chorionic villus sampling for chromosomes at 11 weeks' gestation

☐ D Offer amniocentesis testing for chromosomes at 16 weeks' gestation

☐ E Offer detailed cardiac scanning at 22 weeks' gestation

9.13 In a child with disproportionate short stature, the investigation MOST likely to be helpful diagnostically is which of the following?

☐ A Mutation testing for achondroplasia

☐ B Endocrine testing for growth hormone levels and pituitary function

☐ C A skeletal survey

☐ D Examination of both parents

☐ E Assessment of sitting and standing heights and arm span

Extended Matching Questions

9.14 Theme: Renal complications

A Renal agenesis
B Potter syndrome
C Polycystic kidneys
D Renal artery stenosis
E Renal tumours
F Hypertension
G Horseshoe kidney
H Renal tubular acidosis
I Phaeochromocytoma
J Nephropathy

For each of the following conditions, select the most common renal complication from the list above. Each option may be used once, more than once, or not at all.

☐ 1. Turner syndrome
☐ 2. Beckwith–Wiedemann syndrome
☐ 3. Williams syndrome

9.15 Theme: Karyotypes

A 45,X
B 45,Y
C 46,XX
D 46,XY
E 47,XXY
F 47,XXX
G 47,XYY
H 45,XY,t(14;21)
I 46,XX,t(14;21)
J 46,XX,t(7;20)

For each of the following conditions select the appropriate karyotype from the list above. Each option may be used once, more than once, or not at all.

☐ 1. A normal reciprocal translocation carrier
☐ 2. A girl with Christmas disease (haemophilia B)
☐ 3. A boy with Noonan syndrome

MT–F Answers

9.1   Prader–Willi syndrome: A E

Prader–Willi syndrome causes neonatal hypotonia, with poor neonatal feeding. A low metabolic rate conspires with hyperphagia (caused by hypothalamic dysfunction) to produce severe childhood obesity, which can lead to diabetes mellitus and coronary artery disease at a young age. However, it is a rare disorder, and most childhood obesity is caused by poor diet. Affected individuals have mild to moderate learning disability, although around 10% of adults are in the normal range of intelligence. Hypogonadism leads to reduced fertility in females, and infertility in males.

9.2   Congenital adrenal hyperplasia: A B

Congenital adrenal hyperplasia is an autosomal recessive condition that affects males and females in equal proportions. However, because there is virilisation, females are usually detected at birth. There is a definite excess of females to males at all ages, and this might be due to the deaths of undetected males as a result of salt-wasting crises. This only applies to the most common type, 21-hydroxylase deficiency. Women at risk of bearing affected children take dexamethasone from very early in pregnancy until such time as the fetal status can be determined. The steroids are discontinued unless the fetus is female and affected. The treatment suppresses the endogenous production of steroids, and thus reduces the excess androgens present. Virilisation is prevented in about 80% of cases, and reduced in the remainder. Steroid replacement therapy is lifelong, and needs to be increased in times of illness. There is a single common mutation in the most common type of congenital adrenal hyperplasia, and mutation analysis is available in all types. Thus family carrier testing should be possible. Congenital adrenal hyperplasia is not yet part of the neonatal screening programme in the UK, although it is in several other countries.

9.3   Achondroplasia: D E

Trident hand and pronounced lumbar lordosis are classic features of this condition. The limb shortening in achondroplasia is predominantly rhizomelic (proximal limb, ie femur and humerus most affected). There is an increased risk of hydrocephalus, and this should be monitored for the first 2 years of life. However, most children do not suffer this complication. Madelung is a wrist deformity found in Leri–Weill dyschondrosteosis, and not achondroplasia.

9.4   Neurofibromatosis type 1: All false

While plexiform neurofibromas are present from birth, single neurofibromas develop in adulthood. Lisch nodules are not associated with any ocular defect. DNA analysis is not routinely performed in neurofibromatosis type 1 because mutations are found in only about 75% of affected individuals, and the diagnosis is clinical. About 30% of affected individuals have learning difficulties, although there appear to be specific areas of difficulty in a larger number. Reproductive capacity is normal.

9.5   Karyotyping: A B E

Karyotyping (chromosome analysis) will detect most major structural or copy number defects, such as trisomy 21, or deletions giving rise to developmental delay. It is also helpful in determining the gender of a child with a possible virilising condition such as congenital adrenal hyperplasia. Galactosaemia is an autosomal recessive metabolic disorder which is rarely associated with chromosomal abnormalities. Treacher Collins syndrome is autosomal dominant, and although chromosomal anomalies have occasionally been reported, this is rare, and karyotyping is not indicated.

9.6   Cousin marriages: C D E

Although consanguineous marriages do carry an increased risk of autosomal recessive disorders, the majority of couples will not be affected in this way. There is an observed three-fold increase in neonatal death and significant morbidity in the offspring of consanguineous marriages. No doctor should tell a patient not to have children, but advice can be given on specific risks, and targeted carrier testing can be offered. This could cover the common conditions in the specific race of the couple, plus any known disorders within their family.

Best of Five Answers

9.7   E: 8%

Spinal muscular atrophy is an autosomal recessive disorder. Thus this patient, as the sibling of an affected individual, has a carrier risk of 2 in 3. Her partner, as the uncle of an affected individual, has a 1 in 2 carrier risk. Thus, before testing, the risk to this pregnancy is $2/3 \times 1/2 \times 1/4 = 1/12$, or approximately 8%. The gender of the baby does not change the risks.

9.8   A: Galactosaemia

Galactosaemia is not associated with epilepsy of any nature, and classically presents with poor suck, failure to thrive, bleeding diasthesis and jaundice. Untreated galactosaemia can cause hyperammonaemia, sepsis and shock, which may result in seizures eventually. Rett syndrome in males causes a neonatal encephalopathy that is usually fatal. All the other conditions are associated with seizures, including neonatal.

9.9   D: Collect DNA from the father for testing

Hereditary motor and sensory neuropathy is a heterogeneous disease, with only about 50% of individuals having a duplication of *PMP22*. Several other genes are involved. It is pointless to test a family member before the causative mutation is found in the affected individual. As this is largely an adult-onset disease, a normal neurological examination proves nothing, although an abnormal one may suggest that the child is affected. Predictive testing for adult-onset, untreatable disorders is avoided in children, in part to allow them the choice as to whether or not to be tested. Invasive investigations such as nerve conduction studies on a young child who has no symptoms are not indicated.

9.10 D: Homocystinuria

Marfan syndrome causes lens dislocation, but joints are lax and there is not usually any learning disability. Stickler syndrome is associated with an increased risk of retinal detachment and cataracts, but not lens dislocation. Ehlers–Danlos syndrome (EDS) is not a single diagnosis. EDS type VI is associated with an increased risk of globe rupture, but there are no other ocular phenotypes. Benign familial joint hypermobility is EDS III.

9.11 E: Carrier testing for haemoglobinopathies

The autosomal recessive condition for which this couple are at greatest risk and for which carrier testing is available is β-thalassaemia. Turkish people are not a population with a high carrier risk for cystic fibrosis, and the current rate of detection of mutations in the population is quite low, at around 50% (compared with 90% and 95% in the North European Caucasian and Ashkenazi Jewish populations, respectively). Gaucher's disease is common in the Ashkenazi Jewish population, but not in Turkish people. The married cousins are at no increased risk for chromosomal abnormalities as a result of their consanguinity. They will also be at risk of having a child with any autosomal recessive condition, but undirected carrier testing is impossible. Although familial Mediterranean fever is relatively common in Turkey, there are many mutations, and carrier-status cannot be excluded in an unaffected individual with no family history.

9.12 A: Check her chromosomes, and proceed with routine maternal serum screening and anomaly scanning if they are normal

It is most likely that the sister had straightforward trisomy 21, which bears no recurrence risk for siblings. However, the small possibility that it was translocation Down syndrome cannot be excluded, so her chromosomes should be checked. If they are normal, then she is not at any significantly increased risk compared with background risk, and only routine screening is appropriate. If found to carry a Robertsonian translocation involving chromosome 21, she should be offered fetal karyotyping by chorionic villus sampling or amniocentesis. Her risk is too high to rely on serum screening alone in this situation. It is not appropriate to offer invasive testing by chorionic villus sampling or amniocentesis if she is at no increased risk. The atrioventricular septal defect is very likely to be related to the Down syndrome, and she is unlikely to be at any increased risk for having a child with a cardiac abnormality from any other cause.

9.13 C: A skeletal survey

Although achondroplasia is a common cause of disproportionate short stature, it is not the only one. It can be diagnosed reliably by skeletal survey, as can many other causes. Growth hormone deficiency is not associated with disproportionate short stature. The parents could easily be normal if the condition was a new mutation, autosomal dominant or autosomal recessive. Measuring sitting and standing heights and arm span will confirm the disproportion, but this is unlikely to be helpful otherwise.

EMQ Answers

9.14 Renal complications

1. G: Horseshoe kidney

A 45,XO karyotype is highly associated with horseshoe kidney, and renal ultrasound should be arranged at diagnosis. Hypertension is also a complication, but this is frequently secondary to renal disease.

2. E: Renal tumours

The overall risk of tumours in Beckwith–Wiedemann syndrome is 7.5%, although this is much lower if there is no hemihypertrophy. Wilms' tumour is the most common associated tumour, and risks are greater if there is nephromegaly. Affected children should be offered 3-monthly renal ultrasound screening. Other tumours include hepatoblastoma, neuroblastoma, rhabdomyosarcoma, and all embryonal tumours. These are all very rare, so the individual risk for each is low, but much higher than in unaffected children. There is no proven screening for these tumours, although some centres are offering regular testing of serum α-fetoprotein for hepatoblastomas.

3.　D: Renal artery stenosis

Renal anomalies are found in 17% of patients with Williams syndrome. The most common of these is renal artery stenosis, which is usually mild, and not associated with hypertension. Hypercalcaemia can also lead to renal stone formation. Other arteries, such as coronary and intracranial, can also exhibit stenoses.

9.15　Karyotypes

1.　J: 46,XX,t(7;20)

In contrast to chromosomes 13, 14, 15, 21 and 22, neither chromosome 7 nor chromosome 20 are acrocentric, so this translocation must be a reciprocal one in which segments from each of chromosomes 7 and 20 have been exchanged. This means that, in addition to the normal copies of chromosome 7 and 20, there is a chromosome 7 with a piece of chromosome 20 replacing part of its length, and a chromosome 20 with the corresponding piece of chromosome 7 attached. This leaves 46 chromosomes in total in a balanced reciprocal translocation carrier.

2.　A: 45,X

The most likely explanation for a female fully manifesting an X-linked disease is that she has Turner syndrome. The other possibility, but a less likely one, is that she has normal chromosomes but has unfavourably skewed X chromosome inactivation.

3.　D: 46,XY

The karyotype is usually normal in Noonan syndrome.

10. Haematology and Oncology

Multiple True–False Questions

10.1 Regarding idiopathic thrombocytopenic purpura (ITP) in children:

- [ ] A approximately 80% of children recover spontaneously in 6–8 weeks
- [ ] B Measles, mumps and rubella (MMR) vaccination is contraindicated in children who have previously had an episode of ITP
- [ ] C bone marrow aspiration is recommended before a child is treated with steroids
- [ ] D lymphadenopathy and splenomegaly are common findings
- [ ] E recognised treatment options include intravenous immunoglobulins and steroids

10.2 Which of the following statements about hereditary spherocytosis are correct?

- [ ] A a number of surface protein defects have been identified which lead to red cell membrane instability
- [ ] B haemolysis is predominantly intravascular
- [ ] C palpable splenomegaly is generally not present in children
- [ ] D gallstones are a common complication
- [ ] E inheritance is usually autosomal dominant

10.3 von Willebrand disease (vWD)

- [ ] A is caused by a qualitative or quantitative deficiency of von Willebrand factor
- [ ] B results in a bleeding disorder that is characterised by petechiae
- [ ] C usually has an autosomal recessive mode of inheritance
- [ ] D may be associated with low levels of factor VIII levels
- [ ] E has symptoms that usually improve with desmopressin (1-desamino-8-D-arginine vasopressin [DDAVP]) therapy

10.4 Regarding osteosarcoma,

- [ ] A it is the most common primary bone tumour in children
- [ ] B it is seen most commonly in children under the age of 10 years
- [ ] C it is seen with increased frequency in patients who have been previously treated for retinoblastoma
- [ ] D the distal femur and proximal tibia are the most common sites of primary tumours
- [ ] E the outlook for patients presenting with metastatic disease is now extremely good (> 85% long-term survival)

10.5 High serum levels of α-fetoprotein (AFP) may be found in:

- [ ] A normal neonates
- [ ] B hepatitis
- [ ] C hepatoblastoma
- [ ] D sacrococcygeal teratoma
- [ ] E neuroblastoma

10.6 The following is true of neuroblastoma:

- [ ] A it is most commonly metastatic at presentation
- [ ] B approximately 90% of tumours secrete catecholamines, the metabolites of which are detectable in the urine
- [ ] C infants with large liver metastasis and subcutaneous deposits have a poor prognosis
- [ ] D screening in infancy has been clearly demonstrated to reduce mortality
- [ ] E abdominal masses are typically calcified

Best of Five Questions

10.7 A 5-year-old girl presents with a 2-day history of a widespread petechial rash. She is afebrile and systemically well. Examination is otherwise unremarkable. The following haematological parameters were obtained: haemoglobin 11.5 g/dL (normal range [NR] 11.0–14.0 g/dL); platelets 9×10^9/L (NR 150–400 $\times 10^9$/L; white blood cells 6.7 $\times 10^9$/L (NR 4–11 $\times 10^9$/L); neutrophils 2.1 $\times 10^9$/L (NR 2.0–7.5 $\times 10^9$/L). A blood film is normal other than thrombocytopenia. What is the MOST appropriate initial management?

- [ ] A Conservative management with a repeat blood count after a few days
- [ ] B Treatment with intravenous immunoglobulin
- [ ] C Bone marrow aspiration
- [ ] D Platelet transfusion
- [ ] E Treatment with prednisolone

10.8 A 10-year-old boy is in his second year of treatment for acute lymphoblastic leukaemia (ALL) and is poorly compliant with treatment. He presents with several days of breathlessness, pyrexia and cough. On examination, he has a respiratory rate of 40 breaths/min and oxygen saturations of 86% in air. A chest X-ray shows diffuse interstitial infiltrates. Of the following, which is the MOST important treatment to consider?

☐ A Nebulised ribavirin
☐ B Liposomal amphotericin
☐ C High-dose co-trimoxazole
☐ D Intravenous ganciclovir
☐ E Intravenous immunoglobulin

10.9 A 4-year-old girl presents with a 4-week history of right-sided peri-orbital swelling and proptosis. Systemic examination is unremarkable. Plain X-rays show lytic lesions in the peri-orbital bones, but also in other areas of the skull. The MOST likely diagnosis is:

☐ A Osteosarcoma
☐ B Osteomyelitis
☐ C Langerhans cell histiocytosis
☐ D Metastatic neuroblastoma
☐ E Optic glioma

10.10 A 2-year-old boy presents in the Emergency Department with a cough, coryza and fever. On examination he has a red inflamed throat and mild tachypnoea, and has scanty bilateral basal crackles in his chest. Examination is otherwise unremarkable. He has been previously well, thriving, with no previous history of serious infections. A chest X-ray is unremarkable. His blood count reveals: haemoglobin 11 g/dL (normal range [NR] 11.0–14.0 g/dL) white blood cells 6.1×10^9/L (NR $4–11 \times 10^9$/L); neutrophils 0.6×10^9/L (NR $2.0–7.5 \times 10^9$/L); platelets 231×10^9/L (NR $150–450 \times 10^9$/L). Which of the following is the MOST likely cause for his neutropenia?

☐ A Viral infection
☐ B Gram-negative sepsis
☐ C Congenital cyclical neutropenia
☐ D Kostmann syndrome
☐ E Leukaemia

10.11   A 9-year-old girl is seen in clinic with a 6-month history of worsening headaches. Her mother remarks that she has been drinking excessively, and does not seem to have grown significantly over the past 2 years. On examination she has bilateral optic atrophy, reduced visual acuity and a bitemporal hemianopia. Blood tests reveal a serum sodium of 165 mmol/L (normal range 135–145 mmol/L) Which of the following is the MOST likely diagnosis?

☐ A   Langerhans cell histiocytosis
☐ B   Craniopharyngioma
☐ C   Pituitary adenoma
☐ D   Optic glioma
☐ E   Cerebellar medulloblastoma

10.12   Which ONE of the following haematological abnormalities is NOT commonly seen in children with untreated coeliac disease?

☐ A   Prolonged prothrombin time
☐ B   Howell–Jolly bodies on a peripheral blood film
☐ C   Macrocytic anaemia
☐ D   Microcytic anaemia
☐ E   Red cell fragmentation on a blood film

10.13   A 20-month-old boy presents with pallor. He is the first-born child of healthy Mediterranean parents who are distantly related. His diet consists of cow's milk, fortified cereal and, occasionally, vegetables and red meat. Examination, apart from pallor, is unremarkable. His height and weight are on the 20th centile. The following haematological parameters were obtained: haemoglobin 9.0 g/dL (normal range [NR] 11.0–14.0 g/dL); mean corpuscular / cell volume (MCV) 58 fL (NR 80–94 fL); mean corpuscular haemoglobin (MCH) 20 pg (NR 24–31 pg); mean corpuscular haemoglobin concentration (MCHC) 28 g/dL (NR 32–36 g/dL); platelets 260 × 10^9/L (NR 150–400 × 10^9/L); red blood cell count 5.5 × 10^{12}/L (NR 4–5 × 10^{12}/L). Which one of the following is the MOST likely diagnosis?

☐ A   Iron-deficiency anaemia
☐ B   Sideroblastic anaemia
☐ C   Thalassaemia trait
☐ D   Lead poisoning
☐ E   Anaemia of chronic disorders

Extended Matching Questions

10.14 Theme: Blood and coagulation values

	Hb (g/dL)	Platelets (× 10⁹/L)	Total WCC (× 10⁹/L)	Neutrophils (%)	INR	APTT (s)
Normal range	11.0–14.0	150–400	4–11	30–60	0.6–1.17	28–40
A	10.5	42	10	30	1.10	30
B	12.2	340	6	50	1.02	33
C	6.0	40	15	60	1.15	31
D	7.0	20	2	5	1.10	35
E	18.0	150	18	60	1.30	52
F	10.0	190	5	5	0.99	32
G	10.0	28	15	60	2.50	74

APTT, activated partial thromboplastin time; Hb, haemaglobin; INR, international normalised ratio; WCC, white cell count.

For each patient below, select the appropriate haematological parameters listed above. Each option may be used once, more than once, or not at all.

☐ 1. A 1-year-old girl with haemolytic uraemic syndrome.
☐ 2. A 1-year-old boy with Wiskott–Aldrich syndrome.
☐ 3. A normal 2-day-old newborn baby.

10.15 Theme: Associations with cancer in children

A Beckwith–Wiedemann syndrome
B Neurofibromatosis type 1
C Down syndrome
D Ataxia telangiectasia
E Xeroderma pigmentosum
F Li–Fraumeni syndrome
G von Hippel–Lindau disease

For each of the patients below, select a syndrome/disease from the above list that is closely associated with the condition they suffer from. Each option may be used once, more than once, or not at all.

☐ 1. A 3-year-old girl with an optic glioma.
☐ 2. A 5-year-old boy with a Wilms' tumour.
☐ 3. A 4-year-old girl with rhabdomyosarcoma whose mother has recently been diagnosed with breast cancer.

MT–F Answers

10.1 Idiopathic thrombocytopenic purpura (ITP): A C E

In most cases, ITP in children is a benign, self-limiting disorder that does not require any active medical management. However, it is a diagnosis of exclusion, and other more serious conditions, such as leukaemia and aplastic anaemia, should always be considered. Children with ITP are usually well and other clinical signs such as anaemia, hepatosplenomegaly or significant lymphadenopathy are unusual and warrant further investigation. Serious bleeding is rare, and the majority of cases resolve spontaneously over the course of 6–8 weeks. Children without any significant bleeding symptoms can usually be managed expectantly, regardless of the platelet count. In children with significant bleeding (eg gastrointestinal bleeding or recurrent epistaxis), treatment with either steroids or intravenous immunoglobulins is usually effective. Examination of a peripheral blood film by an experienced haematologist is mandatory in all cases. In clinically atypical cases, or when treatment with steroids is being considered, bone marrow aspiration should also be performed. ITP is reported to occur following MMR vaccination, with an estimated occurrence of 1 in 24 000 vaccinations. However, there is no evidence of vaccine-associated recurrence in children who have developed ITP independently of MMR vaccine. MMR vaccination is therefore not contraindicated in these children. In children who have developed ITP within 6 weeks of their first dose of MMR vaccine, the Committee of Safety of Medicines recommends testing serological immunity to measles, mumps and rubella. MMR vaccination is recommended in children without protective immunity.

10.2 Hereditary spherocytosis: A D E

Hereditary spherocytosis is the most common cause of the hereditary haemolytic anaemias seen in Northern Europe. It is a heterogeneous group of disorders caused by molecular defects in the genes that code for red cell membrane proteins such as spectrin and ankyrin. Such defects lead to an abnormal cytoskeleton, with loss of red cell surface area and consequent spherocytosis. Most children with this condition have palpable splenomegaly, but the severity of anaemia and jaundice is very variable. Haemolysis, and consequently jaundice and anaemia, is typically increased during intercurrent infections. Gallstones, caused by chronic haemolysis, are common and can occur even in young children. Haemolysis is predominantly extravascular, with destruction of the abnormal red cells occurring mainly in the spleen. Splenectomy usually results in complete resolution of symptoms. In most cases the family history, clinical signs and blood film are diagnostic and more sophisticated tests (eg osmotic fragility and red cell membrane protein analysis) are not usually needed.

10.3 von Willebrand disease (vWD): A D E

vWD is classified into at least three types (I, II and III). The most common, type I, accounts for at least 70% of patients with vWD and is caused by a partial deficiency of von Willebrand factor (vWF). Type II, much less common, is due to an abnormally functioning vWF, and type III results from a complete absence of vWF. The majority of vWD cases, therefore, are due to a quantitative rather than a qualitative abnormality of vWF. vWF is a multimeric protein needed for platelet adhesion, and the bleeding seen in vWD is characteristically mucous-membrane bleeding, excess bleeding from surgical or dental procedures, and easy bruising – but not characteristically in the form of petechiae. vWF is also a carrier for factor VIII, and reduced factor VIII levels are found in some patients. vWD is inherited in an autosomal dominant manner. Desmopressin, a synthetic analogue of antidiuretic hormone, acts to release endothelial stores of vWF, and is an effective treatment in patients with mild disease.

10.4 Osteosarcoma: A C D

Primary bone tumours account for approximately 5% of all malignancies in children. Roughly two-thirds of these are osteosarcomas, and one third are Ewing's sarcomas. Both osteosarcoma and Ewing's sarcoma are most common in the second decade of life, to the extent that, in adolescents, bone tumours are the third most common malignancy seen, exceeded only by leukaemias and lymphomas. Osteosarcomas are rare in younger children. The majority of osteosarcomas occur in the metaphyses of long bones, with approximately two-thirds occurring around the knee. By contrast, Ewing's sarcoma commonly arises in the pelvis and in the diaphyses of long bones. There will be evidence of metastatic disease, most commonly in the lungs, at presentation in 10–20% of children with osteosarcoma. Although long-term survival from metastatic disease has improved with intensive multi-agent chemotherapy, it remains in the order of 25–40%. Osteosarcoma is the most common second malignancy seen after retinoblastoma. Children with hereditary bilateral retinoblastoma who are carrying germ-line mutations in the retinoblastoma gene (*RB1*) are at risk, particularly if they have received radiotherapy.

10.5 Increased α-fetoprotein (AFP): A B C D

AFP is a protein that is produced primarily during fetal development. Levels fall from birth, but are higher in neonates than in older children. Age-appropriate reference ranges must therefore be used to decide if levels are abnormally elevated. Very high levels are seen in some malignancies, such as hepatoblastoma, hepatocellular carcinoma and germ-cell tumours (eg sacrococcygeal teratoma). AFP levels can be used to screen for these malignancies and also to monitor disease response to treatment. Regenerating liver tissue, such as seen in hepatitis, may cause an elevated AFP. High levels of AFP may also be seen in patients with ataxia telangiectasia.

10.6   Neuroblastoma: A B E

Neuroblastoma is an embryonal tumour of the sympathetic nervous system. It is the most common extracranial solid tumour seen in children, accounting for 8–10% of childhood malignancies. Unfortunately, more than 50% of affected children have metastatic disease at presentation. Approximately 70% of primary tumours arise in the abdomen and are typically calcified – a radiological feature that is useful in distinguishing them from Wilms' tumours. Infants may present with localised primary disease but bulky metastatic disease in the liver, together with subcutaneous nodules. Such a pattern is classified as stage IVS and is associated with a very favourable outcome despite the metastatic nature of the disease. Indeed, in many such infants the tumour will spontaneously regress, or respond to minimal amounts of chemotherapy. Catecholamines are secreted by 90–95% of these tumours; their metabolites (typically vanillylmandelic acid [VMA] and homovanillic acid [HVA]) can be detected in the urine. Urinary catecholamine metabolites have been used as a means of population screening. Such screening has been shown to pick up a number of asymptomatic tumours and results in an increase in the apparent incidence of neuroblastoma in infancy. However, it has not been shown to improve outcome or overall survival of the screened population, suggesting that screening tends to pick up good-risk tumours that may have spontaneously regressed.

Best of Five Answers

10.7   A: Conservative management with a repeat blood count after a few days

The diagnosis is idiopathic thrombocytopenic purpura (ITP). As discussed in the answer to Question 10.1, in most cases ITP in children is a benign, self-limiting disorder that does not require any active medical management. Children with ITP are usually well, and other clinical signs such as anaemia, hepatosplenomegaly or significant lymphadenopathy are unusual and warrant further investigation.

10.8 C: High-dose co-trimoxazole

Pneumocystis jiroveci (previously known as *Pneumocystis carinii)* is an important opportunistic pathogen in children with chronically suppressed cell-mediated immunity such as those receiving treatment for ALL. Pneumocystis carinii pneumonia (PCP) classically presents with cough, fever, tachypnoea and hypoxia that are disproportionate to the apparent degree of respiratory distress. Chest X-ray may show diffuse bilateral infiltrates, but is normal in many cases. *Pneumocystis* is not easily isolated from expectorated sputum or nasal secretions, and bronchoalveolar lavage may be needed for definitive diagnosis. The treatment of choice is high-dose co-trimoxazole, together with steroids. Children receiving treatment for ALL usually receive co-trimoxazole prophylaxis. If this is taken regularly, the diagnosis of PCP is less likely, but in the question it is noted that the child's compliance is poor.

10.9 C: Langerhans cell histiocytosis (LCH)

Langerhans cell histiocytosis is the term used to refer to a spectrum of disorders characterised by clonal proliferation and accumulation of histiocytes (Langerhans cells), with consequent granuloma formation and tissue destruction. It encompasses, and replaces, previous terms such as histiocytosis X, Hand–Schueller–Christian disease, and eosinophilic granuloma. The clinical manifestations of LCH range from asymptomatic lytic lesions in bones to multi-system disease involving skin, bone, liver, bone marrow, lung, and the hypothalamic–pituitary axis (typically with diabetes insipidus). Bone involvement occurs in approximately 80% of cases, with the skull being the most commonly affected site. This can be asymptomatic or present as a painful swelling. Proptosis is common if the orbit is involved. Plain X-rays typically show lytic or 'punched out' lesions. Skin involvement occurs in approximately 25% of cases, and may manifest as a seborrhoeic or eczematous rash, which typically affects the scalp, post-auricular area, and flexures. Although the other diagnoses listed in the question can present with proptosis, they are unlikely to be associated with lytic lesions in the skull.

10.10 A: Viral infection

All the diagnoses listed can cause neutropenia. The question is asking you to decide which is most likely in this patient. The child is thriving, and reached the age of 2 years without any serious infections, making a significant congenital neutropenia (such as Kostmann syndrome or cyclical neutropenia) unlikely. Although children presenting with leukaemia are often neutropenic, they usually have other abnormalities in the blood count, or other clinical signs (eg hepatosplenomegaly and lymphadenopathy). The absence of such abnormalities does not exclude the diagnosis of leukaemia, but makes it much less likely. Infection is the most common cause of acquired neutropenia. Neutropenia in Gram-negative sepsis is a sign of severe infection in an unwell child. This does not fit with the description of the relatively well child described here. This leaves viral infection as a cause. Not only is this the most common cause of acquired neutropenia in an otherwise well child, but the child's other signs and symptoms support this diagnosis.

10.11   B: Craniopharyngioma

This child's signs and symptoms suggest pathology involving the optic chiasm (bitemporal hemianopia) and pituitary (diabetes insipidus and possible growth hormone deficiency). The fact that she has not grown for 2 years implies long-standing disease. Although answers A to D could all account for disease in this area, in a child of this age craniopharyngioma is the most likely cause. Craniopharyngiomas account for almost 10% of paediatric brain tumours and are usually slowly growing, histologically benign tumours occurring in the sellar or supra-sellar region. This is a classic history of a child with such a tumour; the most common presenting symptoms being nausea, vomiting, headache, and visual disturbance. The majority of patients have evidence of endocrine dysfunction at presentation, typically diabetes insipidus and panhypopituitarism.

10.12   E: Red cell fragmentation on a blood film

Haematological abnormalities are frequently seen in coeliac disease, and may in fact occur in the absence of overt gastrointestinal symptoms. Malabsorption of iron, vitamin B_{12} or folate commonly lead to anaemia, which can be severe. The red cells may indicate macrocytic, microcytic or normocytic anaemia, depending on which deficiency predominates. Malabsorption of vitamin K is also common in untreated disease, and may lead to a coagulopathy. Patients with coeliac disease invariably have a degree of functional hyposplenism, and in many patients this is sufficiently severe to result in blood film abnormalities. Haematological features of hyposplenism include Howell–Jolly bodies (round nuclear remnants seen in red blood cells) and target cells. Red cell fragmentation is a feature of intravascular haemolysis, and would not be an expected finding in a child with coeliac disease.

10.13   C: Thalassaemia trait

This question tests your ability to differentiate the potential causes of microcytic hypochromic anaemia. Iron-deficiency anaemia will be the most common entity in this age group, followed by thalassaemia trait, and the final three causes (sideroblastic anaemia, lead poisoning and anaemia of chronic disorders) will be way down the list. Therefore, to distinguish between iron-deficiency anaemia and thalassaemia trait, the history may be helpful. In this case, if the dietary history is reliable, iron-deficiency anaemia is possible, but not likely. The parents of this patient, being of Mediterranean descent and distantly related, may be carriers of thalassaemia and therefore thalassaemia trait is a definite possibility. The platelet and red blood cell counts are two useful parameters in helping to distinguish iron-deficiency anaemia from thalassaemia trait. The platelet count in iron-deficiency anaemia is normally increased, or is at least at the upper range of normal, whereas the red blood cell count is low. In contrast, the red blood cell count is normally increased in thalassaemia trait, whereas the haemoglobin is low, but not as low as that seen in iron-deficiency anaemia. For the above reasons, the most likely diagnosis would be thalassaemia trait.

EMQ Answers

10.14   Blood and coagulation values

1. C

The haemolytic uraemic syndrome (HUS) occurs throughout the world and is the most common cause of acute renal failure in children in North America and Western Europe. It is characterised by a haemolytic anaemia, thrombocytopenia and renal failure. The most common form occurs in children and is associated with a diarrhoeal illness. Line C in the table has the most appropriate haematological parameters for HUS, in that there is anaemia and thrombocytopenia, with the other parameters being normal. One could confuse lines C and D, but in D there is an associated neutropenia, which is generally not seen in HUS.

2. A

Wiskott–Aldrich syndrome, an X-linked recessive genetic condition, causes persistent thrombocytopenia and in its complete form also causes small platelets, atopy, cellular and humoral immunodeficiencies (particularly immunoglobulin deficiency), and an increased risk of autoimmune disease and haematological malignancies. Line A has the most appropriate haematological parameters for the Wiskott–Aldrich syndrome, in that there is an isolated thrombocytopenia.

3. E

A normal 2-day-old neonate characteristically will have haematological parameters similar to those in line E, in that the haemoglobin is slightly elevated, platelet count is normal, total white cell count is increased relative to an older child, and the INR and APTT are slightly prolonged.

10.15   Associations with cancer in children

1.   B: Neurofibromatosis type 1

Patients with neurofibromatosis type 1 are prone to develop central nervous system gliomas, particularly optic gliomas. These are low-grade or benign tumours, but because of their location can cause significant morbidity and potential mortality.

2.   A: Beckwith–Wiedemann syndrome

The overgrowth syndromes, particularly Beckwith–Weidemann syndrome (macroglossia, organomegaly, omphalos, and hemihypertrophy) are associated with Wilms' tumour and, to a lesser extent, hepatoblastoma. Wilms' tumour is associated with other syndromes, particularly 'WAGR' syndrome (**W**ilms' tumour, **a**niridia, **g**enitourinary abnormalities and mental **r**etardation), Denys–Drash syndrome (pseudohermaphroditism, Wilms' tumour and nephrotic syndrome) and Perlman syndrome (phenotypically similar to Beckwith–Weidemann syndrome).

3.   F: Li–Fraumeni syndrome

Li–Fraumeni is a rare, autosomal dominant, cancer-predisposition syndrome. It is caused by abnormalities in the *p53* tumour suppressor gene. Malignancies can develop in young children, most commonly soft-tissue sarcomas and adrenocortical carcinomas. In adolescents and young adults, there is a greatly increased risk of cancer, including leukaemias, and breast, ovarian, brain and lung carcinomas. Affected individuals often develop second primary tumours.

11. Hepatology

Multiple True–False Questions

11.1 In autoimmune liver disease

- [ ] A the majority of patients have increased serum levels of IgM
- [ ] B more than two-thirds of cases present insidiously
- [ ] C the presence of antibodies to soluble liver antigen (anti-SLA antibodies) is associated with a more severe disease
- [ ] D patients with liver/kidney microsomal type 1 (LKM-1) antibody are more likely to develop acute liver failure
- [ ] E autoimmune sclerosing cholangitis responds poorly to steroid therapy

11.2 Features of Alagille syndrome include:

- [ ] A autosomal dominant inheritance
- [ ] B an audible cardiac murmur in more than 90% of patients
- [ ] C hypercholesterolaemia and hypertriglyceridaemia
- [ ] D growth failure and delayed puberty
- [ ] E extrahepatic biliary hypoplasia

11.3 Which of the following is true of Wilson's disease?

- [ ] A the most common genetic mutation is H1069Q on chromosome 13
- [ ] B neurological symptoms typically present in the first decade of life
- [ ] C Kayser–Fleischer rings are not pathognomonic
- [ ] D serum caeruloplasmin levels may be normal in up to 25% of patients
- [ ] E a hepatic copper concentration < 50 μg/g dry weight of liver rules out the presence of the condition

11.4 In Crigler–Najjar syndrome type I

- [ ] A the mutation occurs in the same gene that is involved in Gilbert syndrome
- [ ] B hepatocyte uptake of bilirubin is abnormal
- [ ] C liver biopsy is normal
- [ ] D inheritance is autosomal dominant
- [ ] E the risk of kernicterus is increased

11.5 Portal hypertension in children

- [ ] A   is most commonly caused by portal vein thrombosis
- [ ] B   occurs when the portal vein to hepatic vein pressure gradient is more than 5 mmHg
- [ ] C   can result in pancytopenia
- [ ] D   is more likely to cause variceal bleeding if the underlying aetiology is at the sinusoidal level
- [ ] E   might not be associated with splenomegaly

11.6 Associations with hepatoblastoma include:

- [ ] A   familial adenomatous polyposis
- [ ] B   prematurity
- [ ] C   Beckwith–Wiedemann syndrome
- [ ] D   Meckel's diverticulum
- [ ] E   trisomy 18

11.7 Causes of neonatal acute liver failure include:

- [ ] A   biliary atresia
- [ ] B   galactosaemia
- [ ] C α_1-antitrypsin deficiency
- [ ] D   herpes simplex virus
- [ ] E   neonatal haemochromatosis

11.8 Liver steatosis can occur with which of the following?

- [ ] A   malnutrition
- [ ] B   total parenteral nutrition
- [ ] C α_1-antitrypsin deficiency
- [ ] D   hepatitis A
- [ ] E   type 1 diabetes mellitus

11.9 It is true of hepatitis A virus that

- [ ] A   it is a DNA virus
- [ ] B   it has an average incubation period of 30 days
- [ ] C   infection can persist for more than 3 months
- [ ] D   it can cause Guillain–Barré syndrome
- [ ] E   infectivity from faecal shedding begins at the onset of symptoms

Best of Five Questions

11.10 A 13-year-old Vietnamese boy had an allogenic bone marrow transplantation performed for relapsed acute lymphoblastic leukaemia. Total body irradiation was administered pre-transplant. Nineteen days after transplantation, he complained of abdominal pain and was noted to be jaundiced. A physical examination showed an increased jugular venous pressure, tender enlarged liver and ascites. His body weight had increased by 3 kg. Laboratory results showed: total bilirubin 143 μmol/L, direct bilirubin 86 μmol/L, alanine aminotransferase (ALT) 356 U/L, aspartate aminotransferase (AST) 408 U/L, alkaline phosphatase (ALP) 268 U/L, γ-glutamyl transpeptidase (γGT) 248 U/L. Doppler ultrasound showed an increase in the hepatic artery resistance index, but hepatic venous flow was normal. What is the MOST likely diagnosis here?

- [ ] A Acute graft-versus-host disease
- [ ] B Veno-occlusive disease
- [ ] C Sepsis
- [ ] D Cytomegalovirus (CMV) hepatitis
- [ ] E Congestive cardiac failure

11.11 A Chinese lady delivers a pre-term baby boy weighing 1.9 kg. She had no documented hepatitis B virus (HBV) screen. Which of the following would be the MOST appropriate plan for the immediate immunisation of her newborn?

- [ ] A No HBV vaccine or anti-HBV immunoglobulin should be given
- [ ] B Give HBV vaccine within 12 hours of birth only
- [ ] C Give anti-HBV immunoglobulin within 12 hours of birth only
- [ ] D Give both HBV vaccine and anti-HBV immunoglobulin within 12 hours of birth if mother's hepatitis B surface antigen (HBsAg) status cannot be determined in that period
- [ ] E Give HBV vaccine within 12 hours, perform a HBsAg test for the mother, and administer anti-HBV immunoglobulin within 7 days if the mother tests positive

11.12 A 10-day-old girl was brought to the Emergency Department because of haematemesis. She is the first child of unrelated parents and was exclusively breast-fed. She had begun to feed less well and started vomiting over the previous 3 days. The baby had woken up at around midnight with difficulties in breathing, and vomited obvious fresh blood repeatedly. Clinical examination revealed a floppy child with bilateral cataracts. The liver was firm and palpable 3 cm below the costal margin, and the spleen was enlarged at 1.5 cm. The initial blood sugar stick measurement was 1.1 mmol/L. Urine dipstick showed blood ++, protein +++, ketones +. Urine reducing sugar was positive. Other investigations revealed: haemoglobin 12.1 g/dL, platelets 103 × 10⁹/L, bilirubin 135 μmol/L, ALT 195 U/L, ammonia 28 μmol/L, lactate 7.6 mmol/L, prothrombin time (PT) 36 s, activated partial thromboplastin time (APTT) 93 s. Blood cultures were performed on admission and returned, 2 days later, positive for *Escherichia coli*. The test(s) MOST likely to clinch the diagnosis of the underlying cause would be:

☐ A Urine succinyl acetone and plasma amino acid assay
☐ B α_1-Antitrypsin level and phenotype
☐ C Liver biopsy for histology, electron microscopy and measurement of electron-chain activities
☐ D Plasma acyl carnitine profile
☐ E Erythrocyte galactose-1-phosphate uridyl transferase levels

11.13 A 7-year-old Indian boy presented with jaundice, abdominal pain, and poor appetite for 2 days. He had returned from India 4 days previously, after spending 1 week in a rural village visiting his relatives. Soon after arriving in India, he developed a fever and skin rash that started from the face, spreading to the trunk. He was being treated with amoxicillin for a throat infection, and the rash had been attributed to amoxicillin allergy. He had his antibiotic changed to clarithromycin and the fever and rash subsided just before he returned to the UK. He had scleral icterus, tender hepatomegaly of 4 cm and splenomegaly of 2 cm, but no significant lymphadenopathy. The urine appeared dark. Laboratory values were: haemoglobin 12.3 g/dL, white blood count 15.9 × 10⁹/L (8% atypical lymphocytes, 20% neutrophils), total bilirubin 87 μmol/L, AST 123 U/L, ALT 256 U/L, ALP 156 U/L. The MOST likely diagnosis is:

☐ A Infectious mononucleosis
☐ B Hepatitis A infection
☐ C Leptospirosis
☐ D Drug-induced liver disease
☐ E Measles

Extended Matching Questions

11.14 Theme: Hepatitis B

	ALT	HBV DNA	cAb	sAg	sAb	eAg	eAb
A	↑	Detectable	IgM	+	–	+	–
B	↑	Detectable	IgM	+	–	–	–
C	↑	Detectable	IgG	+	–	+	–
D	N	High	IgG	+	–	+	–
E	N	Undetectable	IgG	–	+	–	+
F	N	Undetectable	IgG	+	–	–	+

↑, increased; ALT, alanine aminotransferase; cAb, core antibody; eAb, envelope antibody; eAg, envelope antigen; HBV, hepatitis B virus; N, normal; sAb, surface antibody; sAg, surface antigen.

For each of the serologies above, select the correct diagnosis from the following. Each option may be used once, more than once, or not at all.

- [ ] 1. Chronic hepatitis B infection, non-replicative phase.
- [ ] 2. Acute hepatitis B infection with pre-core mutant.
- [ ] 3. Chronic hepatitis B infection, immune clearance phase.

11.15 Theme: Chronic liver disease

A   Alagille syndrome
B   Wilson's disease
C   Chronic hepatitis B infection
D   Autoimmune liver disease
E   Cystic fibrosis liver disease
F α_1-Antitrypsin deficiency
G   Glycogen storage disease
H   Gaucher's disease

For each of the patients below, select the most likely diagnosis from those listed above. Each option may be used once, more than once, or not at all.

☐   1.   A 9-year-old girl presents with a 6-week history of lethargy, decreased appetite, weight loss, and intermittent dark urine and pale stools. She had a similar episode 1 year previously, but was not investigated because she recovered quickly. Clinically, she was jaundiced but alert. A firm liver of 5 cm and a small spleen were palpable. Investigations revealed: total bilirubin 68 μmol/L, direct bilirubin 49 μmol/L, total protein 86 g/L, albumin 30 g/L, ALT 343 U/L, AST 375 U/L, ALP 193 U/L, prothrombin time 16 s, serum caeruloplasmin normal, anti-nuclear antibodies (ANA) negative, α_1-antitrypsin phenotype PiMM.

☐   2.   A 5-year-old Chinese boy is being investigated for marked hepatomegaly extending to the level of the umbilicus. His height is 90 cm and his weight is 11.3 kg (both below the 3rd centile). Investigations revealed: total protein 84 g/L, albumin 49 g/L, total bilirubin 19 μmol/L, ALP 282 U/L, ALT 64 U/L, AST 78 U/L, γGT 28 U/L, prothrombin time 12 s, α-fetoprotein 2.2 μg/L, uric acid 467 μmol/L (normal range 130–390 μmol/L), fasting glucose 2.3 mmol/L, fasting triglycerides 3.44 g/L (normal range 0.31–1.08 g/L).

☐   3.   A 14-year-old Pakistani boy presents with jaundice and a change in behaviour. He was aggressive and non-co-operative during examination. Spider naevi, palmar erythema, and a hepatomegaly of 3 cm were observed. Laboratory investigations revealed: haemoglobin 8.3 g/dL, reticulocytes 3%, direct Coombs' test (DCT) negative, total bilirubin 328 μmol/L, ALT 72 U/L, AST 316 U/L, ALP 197 U/L, urine protein ++, urine sugar +.

MT–F Answers

11.1 Autoimmune liver disease: C D

Autoimmune liver disease comprises three forms:

- autoimmune hepatitis
- autoimmune sclerosing cholangitis
- de-novo autoimmune hepatitis after liver transplant.

Autoimmune hepatitis (AIH) has a 75% female preponderance. Twenty percent of patients have other associated autoimmune diseases. The majority of cases present like an acute viral hepatitis (50% smooth muscle antibody (SMA)/ANA +ve; 65% LKM-1 +ve); other cases present either insidiously with relapsing jaundice, headache, anorexia and weight loss (38% SMA/ANA +ve; 25% LKM-1 +ve), or are asymptomatic until the complications of portal hypertension set in. Disease is classified on the basis of auto-antibodies:

- type 1:   SMA/ANA +ve
- type 2:   LKM-1 +ve.

The presence of anti-SLA antibody is associated with a more severe disease, whereas patients who are LKM-1 +ve are more likely to develop acute liver failure. Up to 20% of patients with AIH do not have auto-antibodies detectable at presentation. In 80% of patients, IgG levels will also be increased.

Autoimmune sclerosing cholangitis (ASC) is an uncommon disorder characterised by chronic inflammation and fibrosis of the bile ducts. It can overlap with AIH; 40% of patients with ASC have clinical, biochemical, immunological and histological features similar to those of AIH. Perinuclear anti-neutrophil cytoplasmic antibodies are found more often in ASC (74%) than in AIH (36%). Inflammatory bowel disease has been found to be present in 44% of children with cholangiopathy, compared with 18% of those with typical AIH. Unlike adult primary sclerosing cholangitis, there is a good response to steroids.

Treatment of autoimmune liver disease (without liver failure) is with prednisolone (starting dose 2 mg/kg per day; maximum dose 60 mg). A maximum of 2 mg/kg per day of azathioprine can be added for better disease control or steroid sparing.

11.2 Alagille syndrome: A B C D

Alagille syndrome or arteriohepatic dysplasia is dominantly inherited with variable penetration. It occurs in 1 in 100 000 live births and results from the mutation of the *JAG1* gene on chromosome 20p12. Diagnosis is made clinically on the basis of chronic cholestasis from intrahepatic biliary hypoplasia, characteristic facies (broad forehead, deep-set eyes, mild hypertelorism, small chin), cardiac murmur, vertebral anomalies, and the presence of posterior embryotoxon. A cardiac murmur can be auscultated at some time in 95% of patients. The pulmonary vascular tree is usually involved, with peripheral pulmonary artery stenosis as the main lesion. Other cardiac lesions include tetralogy of Fallot, truncus arteriosus, secundum atrial septal defect (ASD), patent ductus arteriosus (PDA), ventricular septal defect (VSD) and pulmonary atresia. Intrauterine growth retardation and failure to thrive, with severe malnutrition, occur in 50% of those affected. Other features include renal disease, delayed puberty or hypogonadism, mental retardation, learning difficulties or psychosocial dysfunction, vascular abnormalities, hypothyroidism and pancreatic insufficiency, recurrent otitis media, chest infection, and hypercholesterolaemia. The phenotype is variable. Severe liver disease may require liver transplantation.

11.3 Wilson's disease: A C D E

Wilson's disease has an autosomal recessive inheritance (incidence 1 in 50 000) and results from a mutation of the *ATP7B* gene on chromosome 13q14.3 (most commonly, H1069Q). Clinical presentation can be hepatic (5–12 years), neurological (second decade) or asymptomatic (detected at family screening). Others signs include sunflower-shaped cataracts, acute haemolytic anaemia and renal, cardiac or skeletal abnormalities. The diagnosis is suggested by:

Diagnostic signs	Pitfalls
• Low serum copper	Plasma copper may be normal or raised from hepatic necrosis
• Low plasma caeruloplasmin (< 200 mg/L)	Plasma caeruloplasmin levels exceed 200 mg/L in about 5–25% of cases
	Elevated levels are also seen with oestrogen therapy, infection, inflammation and pregnancy
	Decreased levels are seen with malnutrition, protein-losing enteropathy, nephrotic syndrome, hepatic insufficiency, neonates, Menkes syndrome, hereditary hypocaeruloplasminaemia, heterozygosity for Wilson's disease

continued on next page

• Raised urinary copper (> 25 μmol/24 h)	Poor sensitivity and specificity, greater discrimination after penicillamine challenge. In presymptomatic and some symptomatic cases, post-penicillamine levels may not reach 25 μmol/24 h
	Urinary copper can be raised in other liver diseases
	Difficulties in collecting 24–hour urine samples, especially in smaller children
• Raised liver copper (> 250 μg/g dry weight of liver)	Levels can also be raised in normal infants younger than 6 months, cholestasis syndromes, biliary atresia, paucity of intrahepatic ducts, sclerosing cholangitis, primary biliary cirrhosis, Indian childhood cirrhosis, primary hepatic tumours
	Normal hepatic copper (< 50 μg/g dry weight of liver) rules out Wilson's disease
• Mutation analysis	Many mutations are now known, the most common being H1069Q. However, many patients are compound heterozygotes and different molecular strategies need to be adopted for different populations

Kayser–Fleischer rings are not pathognomonic of Wilson's disease, and can also be found in chronic active hepatitis, primary biliary cirrhosis, cryptogenic cirrhosis, and any intrahepatic cholestasis with cirrhosis. Treatment is with penicillamine 20 mg/kg per day (gradually increased from 5 mg/kg per day) and pyridoxine 10 mg/week. Other drugs that can be used include triethylene tetramine dihydrochloride (trientine), zinc sulphate or zinc acetate, and tetrathiomolybdate. Liver transplantation may be required for fulminant hepatic failure.

11.4   Crigler–Najjar syndrome type I: A C E

Inherited unconjugated hyperbilirubinaemia is a spectrum of disease that depends on the degree of bilirubin uridine diphosphate glucuronosyl transferase (UGT) deficiency caused by mutation of the *UGT1A1* gene. Liver function tests and histology are normal. The spectrum comprises:

- Gilbert syndrome (GS)
- Crigler–Najjar type I
- Crigler–Najjar type II.

Inheritance is autosomal recessive. Gilbert syndrome and Crigler–Najjar syndrome type II can also have autosomal dominant transmission.

   Gilbert syndrome is characterised by a mild deficiency (≥ 50% decrease in UGT activity) and occurs in 7% of the population. It usually presents after puberty, with an incidental finding of increased bilirubin on blood tests, or jaundice after a period of fasting or intercurrent illness. It is more common in males. It is polymorphic for chromosome 2q37: TA repeats in the promoter region (TATA box) in white populations, compared with exon mutations in Asian populations. Correlations between hepatic enzyme activity and serum bilirubin levels are unpredictable, as up to 40% of patients with Gilbert syndrome (and of those with Crigler–Najjar syndrome type II) have a decreased red blood cell lifespan. There is a higher incidence of neonatal jaundice and breast milk jaundice. No treatment is required, and the syndrome is compatible with a normal lifespan.

Two forms of **Crigler–Najjar syndrome** are recognised:

- Type I   Severe deficiency of UGT
  High risk of kernicterus
  Affected individuals require lifelong phototherapy, or even liver transplantation (auxiliary or orthotopic)
- Type II   Moderate deficiency
  May require phototherapy and phenobarbital.

11.5   Portal hypertension in children: C D E

Portal hypertension is defined as portal vein pressure > 5 mmHg or a portal vein to hepatic vein pressure gradient > 10 mmHg. Features include splenomegaly with resultant hypersplenism (thrombocytopenia, anaemia, leukopenia), oesophageal, gastric and rectal varices, ascites and encephalopathy. Splenomegaly can be absent if there are associated splenic malformations (eg asplenia, polysplenia situs inversus), especially in biliary atresia, a common cause of portal hypertension. Portal hypertension and variceal bleeding are major causes of morbidity and mortality (30–50%) in children. They most commonly result from liver cirrhosis, although causes may also be at the pre-sinusoidal level (eg portal vein thrombosis) or the post-sinusoidal level (eg Budd–Chiari disease, veno-occlusive disease). Management is aimed at the prevention and control of oesophageal variceal bleeding. Sclerotherapy, endoscopic variceal ligation, surgical porto-systemic shunts, transjugular intrahepatic porto-systemic shunt (TIPS), oesophageal transection and devascularisation, and pharmacotherapy (eg propranolol and octreotide) are some measures that can be employed.

11.6   Associations with hepatoblastoma: All true

Hepatoblastoma accounts for 79% of liver cancers in children. Males are more frequently affected. It originates from immature liver precursor cells and is usually unifocal and in the right lobe. Metastases to the lungs and central nervous system are common. Hepatoblastoma normally presents in children younger than 3 years with an abdominal mass. Disease is already advanced in 40% of patients at diagnosis, and 20% may have pulmonary metastases. More rare presentations include acute abdomen from tumour rupture, hemihypertrophy and precocious puberty. Hepatoblastoma is associated with familial adenomatous polyposis, prematurity, Beckwith–Wiedemann syndrome, Meckel's diverticulum, trisomy 18, cardiac malformations (patent ductus arteriosus, tetralogy of Fallot), renal abnormalities (dysplasia, horseshoe kidney), extrahepatic biliary atresia, Goldenhar syndrome, and Prader–Willi syndrome. Diagnosis is aided by:

- calcifications on plain radiographs and ultrasound of the liver
- raised platelet count from increased thrombopoietin
- raised α-fetoprotein (80% of patients)
- magnetic resonance imaging or computed tomography scan with intravenous contrast.

Tumours that can be completely resected and have pure fetal-pattern histology have the best prognosis. Cisplatin is the most active single-agent chemotherapy, but combinations may be required.

11.7 Neonatal acute liver failure: B D E

Acute liver failure is the final common pathway of a variety of insults to the liver. Causes vary with age group, and knowledge of the possible aetiologies helps in narrowing down the differential diagnoses, allowing more focused investigations, earlier diagnosis, and specific treatments. Causes of neonatal acute liver failure include perinatal herpes simplex virus infection, neonatal haemochromatosis, galactosaemia, tyrosinaemia, haemophagocytic lymphohistiocytosis, septicaemia, mitochondrial cytopathies, congenital disorders of glycosylation, and severe birth asphyxia. Treatment of acute liver failure remains supportive, unless there is a specific measure for the diagnosis, eg aciclovir for herpes simplex virus infection, 2-(2-nitro-4-trifluoromethylbenzoyl)-1,3-cyclohexanedione (NTBC; Nitisinone) for hereditary tyrosinaemia, iron chelation and antioxidant cocktail for neonatal haemochromatosis.

11.8 Liver steatosis: A B C E

Abnormal accumulation of lipids, usually triglycerides, within the cytoplasm of hepatocytes, either as multiple small droplets or as a single large droplet, can result from many disease processes. Primary fatty liver disease comprises non-alcoholic fatty liver disease (NAFLD) and non-alcoholic steatohepatitis (NASH):

- NAFLD is simple steatosis with no inflammation or scarring, and is benign and reversible.
- NASH occurs when hepatic steatosis results in hepatic inflammation. It can ultimately lead to cirrhosis, liver failure, and hepatocellular carcinoma. Obesity and type 2 diabetes mellitus are associated. Insulin resistance and lipid peroxidation are believed to be involved in the pathogenesis.

Secondary fatty liver disease can result from chronic liver conditions such as hepatitis B, hepatitis C, Wilson's disease, haemochromatosis, α_1-antitrypsin deficiency, autoimmune liver disease, cystic fibrosis and drug toxicity (eg valproate, tetracycline, asparaginase). Disturbances in carbohydrate, protein and lipid metabolism (eg steroid therapy, malnutrition, parenteral nutrition, galactosaemia, hereditary fructose intolerance, glycogen storage disease, tyrosinaemia, homocystinuria, mitochondrial oxidation and respiratory chain defect, Reye syndrome, cholesterol ester storage disease, abetalipoproteinaemia) may also contribute.

11.9   Hepatitis A virus: B C D

Hepatitis A is the most common form of acute viral hepatitis, accounting for 20–25% of all clinically apparent hepatitis worldwide. The RNA virus is spread via the orofaecal route. The incubation period is 2–6 weeks. Infectivity from faecal shedding begins during the prodromal phase, peaks at the onset of symptoms, and then declines rapidly. Shedding may persist for up to 3 months. Hepatitis A is usually asymptomatic; fewer than 5% of infected people have an identifiable illness. Symptomatic infection increases with age at the time of acquisition. Mortality is 0.2–0.4% of symptomatic cases, and is increased in individuals older than 50 or younger than 5 years. Morbidity and mortality are associated with fulminant hepatic failure, prolonged cholestasis, recurrent hepatitis, and extrahepatic complications such as:

- neurological involvement: Guillain–Barré, syndrome, transverse myelitis, post-viral encephalitis, mononeuritis multiplex
- renal disease: acute interstitial nephritis, mesangioproliferative glomerulonephritis, nephrotic syndrome, acute renal failure
- acute pancreatitis
- autoimmune haemolytic anaemia.

Best of Five Answers

11.10 B: Veno-occlusive disease

Abnormal liver function occurs in about 30% of patients undergoing bone marrow transplantation. Common potential causes include infections, graft-versus-host disease (GVHD), veno-occlusive disease and drug toxicity. Veno-occlusive disease is characterised by the triad of jaundice, tender hepatomegaly and weight gain (2–5%). It usually occurs in the first 3 weeks after bone marrow transplantation. Predisposing factors include pre-transplant viral hepatitis, radiotherapy, or busulfan conditioning. There may be an increase in hepatic artery resistance index, but reversed hepatic venous blood flow occurs late in the disease. Treatment includes careful management of fluid status and thrombolytic therapy.

Acute GVHD usually occurs in recipients of allogenic bone marrow transplants 7–50 days after transplant, corresponding to the timing of engraftment. It usually occurs in several systems, commonly including skin and intestine. Liver biopsy may show bile duct damage, lymphocyte infiltrates, and cholestasis, resembling hepatitis C virus infection. Treatment is to increase immunosuppression.

11.11 D: Give both HBV vaccine and anti-HBV immunoglobulin within 12 hours of birth if mother's hepatitis B surface antigen (HBsAg) status cannot be determined in that period

This baby is representative of a high-risk group that requires immediate treatment instead of waiting for results. Women admitted for delivery without documentation of HBsAg test results should have blood drawn and tested as soon as possible after admission. While test results are pending, all infants born to women without documentation of HBsAg test results should receive the first dose of single-antigen hepatitis B vaccine (without hepatitis B immunoglobulin) within 12 hours of birth. If the mother tests HBsAg-positive, her infant should also receive hepatitis B immunoglobulin (HBIg) as soon as possible, but no later than age 7 days. All infants should complete a total of three doses of vaccine. There is potentially decreased immunogenicity of vaccine in pre-term infants weighing less than 2000 g. These infants should receive both single-antigen hepatitis B vaccine and HBIg if the mother's HBsAg status cannot be determined within 12 hours of birth. The birth dose of vaccine should not be counted as part of the three doses required to complete the vaccine series: three additional doses of vaccine (for a total of four doses) should be administered.

11.12 E: Erythrocyte galactose-1-phosphate uridyl transferase levels

Galactosaemia is an autosomal recessive disorder caused by a deficiency of galactose-1-uridyl transferase. An infective and/or metabolic process is the most likely underlying cause. However, Gram-negative sepsis (usually *Escherichia coli*) can be associated, and the clinical picture of sepsis and coagulopathy can be so overwhelming that the underlying metabolic cause is missed (as was the case in this patient). Infants may present with collapse, hypoglycaemia, encephalopathy, vomiting, diarrhoea, jaundice, liver failure, severe coagulopathy, renal tubular dysfunction and cataracts. Clinical assessment should concentrate on resuscitation before a complete history and physical examination are done. Intercurrent illnesses that may have precipitated the metabolic episode must be ruled out. Until the diagnosis is confirmed, management is supportive (correct hypoglycaemia, coagulopathy, acid-base and electrolyte abnormalities; give empirical broad-spectrum antibiotic cover). The presence of urinary reducing substance without glycosuria is suggestive, but not diagnostic of galactosaemia. Diagnosis should be confirmed by demonstration of reduced enzyme activity in blood. Galactose must be eliminated from the diet for life.

11.13 A: Infectious mononucleosis

This child presents with clinical features of acute hepatitis. Differential diagnoses include:

- infections
- drug-induced hepatitis
- metabolic disorders
- autoimmune liver disease.

Infectious mononucleosis is the most likely diagnosis, as there was a history of pharyngitis, a rash after amoxicillin, and there were atypical lymphocytes. Confirmation is with antibody to Epstein–Barr viral capsid antigen (EBV VCA IgM and IgG). Although hepatitis A is a common infection acquired from travels to the developing world, symptoms usually become evident after an incubation period of 2–6 weeks (average 30 days), as shown in the graph on the next page.

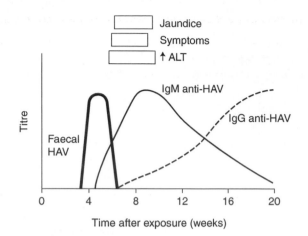

Time after exposure (weeks)

Only 40% of children between 6 and 14 years of age will become jaundiced with hepatitis A virus infection. Transaminase levels are usually much higher in these individuals, with peak ALT 20–100 times the upper limit. In leptospirosis – a spirochaete infection acquired from contaminated water – jaundice usually occurs at the height of fever. In measles, hepatic dysfunction is usually subclinical. Drug-induced liver disease is always a diagnosis of exclusion.

EMQ Answers

11.14 Hepatitis B

1. F
2. B
3. C

Hepatitis B is a DNA hepadnavirus with a worldwide prevalence of 5% (chronic carriers). It is now more commonly acquired vertically from HBeAg-positive mothers (70–90% risk). Horizontal transmission is via parenteral, sexual or environmental sources. Symptomatic acute hepatitis completely resolves in 90% of cases, conferring lifelong immunity. Progression to chronic liver disease can result in cirrhosis and hepatocellular carcinoma. However, chronic infection can be asymptomatic. Asymptomatic chronic infection (HBsAg-positive for at least 6 months) has three phases: immune tolerance, immune clearance, and residual non-replicative.

The following phases of hepatitis B virus infection are recognised:

Host HBV status	ALT	HBV DNA	cAb	sAg	sAb	eAg*	eAb
Acute	↑	Detectable	IgM then IgG	+	–	+	–
Chronic							
Immune tolerance	N	High	IgG	+	–	+	–
Immune clearance	↑	Detectable	IgG	+	–	+	–
Non-replicative	N	Undetectable	IgG	+	–	–	+
Resolved	N	Undetectable	IgG	–	+	–	+

*eAg absent in pre-core mutant. ↑, increased; ALT, alanine aminotransferase; cAb, core antibody; eAb, envelope antibody; eAg, envelope antigen; HBV, hepatitis B virus; N, normal; sAb, surface antibody; sAg, surface antigen.

Clues to remembering:

Hep Bc IgM +ve	Acute infection
Hep Bc IgG +ve with HBsAg +ve	Chronic infection
Presence of HBeAg	Infective and therefore absent in non-replicative and resolved states (except when there is a pre-core mutant)
Abnormal liver function tests	Only occurs during acute infections and clearance of virus

HBeAg, hepatitis B envelope antigen; HBsAg, hepatitis B surface antigen; Hep Bc, hepatitis B virus core antigen.

Experience in treating hepatitis B is limited in paediatrics. Immunomodulation (interferon [IFN]-α, pegylated interferon) and/or antiviral drugs (lamivudine, famciclovir, adefovir) are used. Liver transplantation is indicated for fulminant HBV disease, chronic liver disease and hepatocellular carcinoma. Some children spontaneously clear their chronic infection.

11.15 Chronic liver disease

1. D: Autoimmune liver disease

A female with anorexia, weight loss, relapsing jaundice, and high serum globulin (total protein minus albumin) makes this the best choice for diagnosis. Although ANA is negative, autoimmune liver disease is still top of the list as the diagnosis, as other antibodies such as anti-liver/kidney microsomal (LKM-1) antibody or anti soluble liver antigen (SLA) antibody may be present instead. Up to 20% of patients may not have auto-antibodies detectable at presentation. In 80% of patients, IgG levels will also be raised.

2. G: Glycogen storage disease

Isolated hepatomegaly, failure to thrive, mildly increased plasma aminotransferases, low fasting blood sugar, hyperuricaemia, and hypercholesterolaemia are typical findings in a child with glycogen storage disease type I. Other features include doll-like facies, raised blood lactate, and normal plasma bilirubin, albumin and coagulation.

3. B: Wilson's disease

Signs of chronic liver disease, neuropsychiatric symptoms, Coombs-negative haemolytic anaemia and renal tubular abnormalities in a teenager suggest the diagnosis of Wilson's disease. AST is significantly more increased than ALT, although transaminases and ALP are relatively low. Low serum copper and serum caeruloplasmin, and increased urinary and liver copper will further support this diagnosis. Mutation analysis can now be done. Screening for Kayser–Fleischer rings may be helpful, but these are not pathognomonic for Wilson's disease.

12. Immunology

Multiple True–False Questions

12.1 Immunoglobulin molecules

- [ ] A comprise heavy and light chains
- [ ] B can undergo somatic hypermutation
- [ ] C mediate agglutination
- [ ] D recognise a specific epitope
- [ ] E are part of the innate immune system

12.2 Human T lymphocytes

- [ ] A encode antigen-specific receptors
- [ ] B express class I MHC (major histocompatibility complex) molecules
- [ ] C express immunoglobulin receptors
- [ ] D mediate graft rejection
- [ ] E are targeted by HIV-1

12.3 It is true that placental transfer of antibody

- [ ] A is mediated by Fc receptors?
- [ ] B is complete by 36 weeks of gestation?
- [ ] C protects the newborn against respiratory syncytial virus (RSV)?
- [ ] D can cause heart block?
- [ ] E is reduced in teenage pregnancies?

12.4 Ataxia telangiectasia

- [ ] A is due a mutation of the X chromosome
- [ ] B is associated with IgA deficiency
- [ ] C usually presents at birth
- [ ] D can be cured by bone marrow transplantation
- [ ] E is associated with haematological malignancy

12.5 Type IV hypersensitivity occurs in which of the following?

- [ ] A haemolytic disease of the newborn
- [ ] B contact dermatitis
- [ ] C acute anaphylaxis
- [ ] D disseminated intravascular coagulation
- [ ] E reaction to tuberculin

12.6   Which statements are correct concerning chronic granulomatous disease?

☐ A X-linked inheritance is most common
☐ B it arises as a result of a failure of neutrophil superoxide production
☐ C it is associated with invasive aspergillosis
☐ D it is associated with *Staphylococcus aureus* infections
☐ E neutropenia is characteristic

12.7   In hyper-IgM syndrome,

☐ A inheritance is autosomal dominant
☐ B there is a failure of antibody class switching
☐ C CD4 expression is absent
☐ D there is a strong association with *Cryptosporidium* infections
☐ E liver disease is common

Best of Five Questions

12.8   Which of the following would be MOST suitable to target tumour necrosis factor (TNF) in the management of juvenile idiopathic arthritis?

☐ A Rituximab
☐ B Infliximab
☐ C Trastuzumab (Herceptin)
☐ D Palivizumab
☐ E Imatinib

12.9   A 6-month-old-boy is investigated for failure to thrive. He has severe napkin candidiasis, and a 6-week history of diarrhoea. Full blood count reveals profound lymphopenia. Which is the MOST appropriate investigation?

☐ A Sweat test
☐ B Lymphocyte subset analysis
☐ C Bone marrow examination
☐ D Abdominal computed tomography scan
☐ E Urine culture

12.10 In which one of the following is immunoglobulin therapy of PROVEN benefit?

☐ A Multiple sclerosis
☐ B Chronic granulomatous disease
☐ C Rheumatoid arthritis
☐ D Rheumatic fever
☐ E Kawasaki disease

12.11 An infant is born to an HIV-infected mother in the UK. Which of the following is the MOST appropriate initial action?

☐ A Administer high-dose co-trimoxazole
☐ B Commence triple therapy
☐ C Tell the mother to avoid breast-feeding
☐ D Immunise the infant with BCG
☐ E Administer high-dose immunoglobulin

12.12 A 14-year-old boy undergoes a course of intensive chemotherapy. He is known to be seronegative for herpes zoster. He is visited by his sister, who develops chickenpox the next day. What would the MOST appropriate action be?

☐ A To start oral aciclovir immediately
☐ B To start intravenous aciclovir immediately
☐ C To administer zoster immune globulin within 48 hours
☐ D To suspend his chemotherapy programme and observe
☐ E To observe, and administer zoster immune globulin if lesions develop

12.13 Which of the following is the MOST effective treatment for chronic hepatitis C infection?

☐ A Interferon-α and ribavirin
☐ B Ribavirin alone
☐ C Interferon-γ alone
☐ D Lamivudine alone
☐ E Interferon-α and lamivudine

Extended Matching Questions

12.14 Theme: UK vaccination schedule

A Birth
B 1 month
C 2 months
D 3 months
E 4 months
F 6 months
G 12 months
H Around 2 years
I Around 4 years
J Around 10 years

For the immunisations below, select the most likely timing from the list above. Each option may be used once, more than once, or not at all.

☐ 1. Hepatitis B immunisation if the mother is a known carrier.
☐ 2. MMR vaccination in a child with a family history of Crohn's disease.
☐ 3. The 5-in-1 vaccine.

12.15 Theme: Immune cells

A B cells
B CD4 T cells
C CD8 T cells
D Natural killer cells
E Haematopoietic stem cells
F Mast cells
G Macrophages
H Neutrophils
I Basophils
J Dendritic cells

For the descriptions below, select the most likely cell type from the list above. Each option may be used once, more than once, or not at all.

☐ 1. The population of cells usually reduced or absent in X-linked agammaglobulinaemia.
☐ 2. The cells capable of most effective antigen presentation.
☐ 3. Cells capable of memory response and the direct clearance of virally infected cells.

MT–F Answers

12.1   Immunoglobulin molecules: A B C D

Immunoglobulin molecules mediate agglutination. They are made up of two heavy and two light chains, and the molecule is further subdivided into the variable and constant regions. The variable region, made up of heavy and light chains, binds a specific epitope. Somatic hypermutation is a mechanism that allows continuing diversification of the antibody repertoire through continued mutation of the variable region genes in response to infections. Immunoglobulin production (or humoral immunity) is part of the adaptive, not the innate, immune response.

12.2   T lymphocytes: A B D E

Most T cells develop in the thymus and express the CD3 molecule along with an antigen-specific T-cell receptor that comprises an α and a β chain. As with immunoglobulin molecules, there are constant and variable domains, and diversity is generated by rearrangements of T-cell receptor genes. T cells recognise antigen peptides in association with MHC molecules on the surface of antigen-presenting cells. CD4-expressing helper cells bind to class II MHC and CD8 T cells bind class I MHC. T cells also express MHC class I, and if activated, may also express class II MHC. They are key mediators of graft rejection and graft-versus-host disease.

12.3   Placental transfer of antibody: A C D

IgG crosses the placenta because of active transport of the molecule following interaction between the Fc portion of the molecule and the placental syncytiotrophoblast. The majority of placental transfer occurs in the third trimester and continues until delivery. One major benefit of such antibody transfer is protection against viral pathogens such as RSV in the first months of life. Rarely, antibodies crossing the placenta can have harmful effects, eg heart block can arise in infants of mothers known to have anti-SSA/Ro and/or anti-SSB/La antibodies (the infant may also have transient lupus dermatitis, and hepatic and haematological abnormalities).

12.4   Ataxia telangiectasia: B E

Ataxia telangiectasia usually presents with ataxia or progressive neurological signs; oculocutaneous telangiectasia occurs in children over the age of 2 years. The gene for the disorder (*ATM*) maps to chromosome 11. There is an associated immunodeficiency and IgA levels are often low or absent. Other associations include a high risk of malignancy, growth retardation and liver dysfunction. There is currently no role for transplantation.

12.5 Type IV hypersensitivity: B E

Examples of T-cell-mediated/delayed or type IV hypersensitivity include contact dermatitis, drug reactions, graft-versus-host disease and tuberculin reactivity.

Type	Mediated by	Occurs in
Type I hypersensitivity (immediate)	IgE	Anaphylaxis Atopy Allergy
Type II hypersensitivity (cytotoxic)	IgM and IgG	Haemolytic disease of the newborn Autoimmune haemolytic anaemia Transfusion reactions Hyperacute graft rejection
Type III hypersensitivity	Immune complexes	Arthus reaction Serum sickness
Type IV hypersensitivity (delayed)	T lymphocytes	Delayed-type hypersensitivity Contact sensitivity Tuberculin reaction Graft-versus-host disease

12.6 Chronic granulomatous disease: A B C D

X-linked chronic granulomatous disease is a rare genetic immunodeficiency caused by mutations in the *CYBB* gene, encoding the gp91^{phox} subunit of reduced nicotinamide dinucleotide phosphate (NADPH) oxidase. Diagnosis is based on demonstrating failure of superoxide function in neutrophils (nitroblue tetrazolium test [NBT]). The number of circulating neutrophils is usually normal. Defective phagocyte function results in recurrent bacterial and fungal infections, which can be life-threatening complications. Haematopoietic stem-cell transplantation can cure chronic granulomatous disease, but is generally only considered if a fully HLA-matched donor is available. Gene therapy trials are in progress as an alternative.

12.7 Hyper-IgM syndrome: B D E

In hyper-IgM syndrome, the level of immunoglobulin M (IgM) is usually increased or relatively normal and other immunoglobulin classes are reduced, because cells fail to class switch after exposure to antigen. The most common form is the result of deficiency or absence of CD40 ligand on T cells (so T cells fail to interact with B cells) and is X-linked (Xq26). Infection with *Cryptosporidium* are common, as are sclerosing cholangitis and liver disease.

Best of Five Answers

12.8   B: Infliximab

Infliximab is a monoclonal antibody (mAb) against TNF and has been shown to be of benefit in rheumatoid arthritis, inflammatory bowel disease, and other inflammatory conditions. Rituximab is a mAb against CD20 (on B cells) and is used for certain B-cell malignancies and autoimmune disorders in which B-cell depletion is helpful. Palivizumab targets respiratory syncytial virus (RSV) and is of some benefit in preventing RSV in vulnerable infants (cardiac patients, immunodeficient individuals). Herceptin targets breast cancer oncogene proteins. Imatinib is a tyrosine kinase inhibitor (not a mAb), and is used in chronic myeloid leukaemia to inhibit the *BCR/ABL* oncogene.

12.9   B: Lymphocyte subset analysis

A low lymphocyte count (certainly if below 1.5×10^9/L) in the context of failure to thrive and fungal infection should prompt further investigations. The most useful from the list would be a lymphocyte subset profile. Reduced or absent T cells would suggest severe combined immunodeficiency, which would require immediate therapy with immunoglobulin and a search for bone marrow donors. There may be other reasons for this presentation, such as current infection causing marrow suppression, but severe combined immunodeficiency syndrome (SCID) should be excluded.

12.10 E: Kawasaki disease

Purified IgG in the form of intravenous immunoglobulin is used as replacement therapy in immunodeficiencies and to modify diseases such as Kawasaki disease, in which it has been proved to reduce the incidence of coronary artery aneurysm formation (if used promptly). It has a number of unproven uses, for a variety of different diseases in which its efficacy has not been established.

12.11 C: Tell the mother to avoid breast-feeding

In the UK, the current guidelines recommend treatment of infants of HIV-positive mothers with zidovudine (AZT) from birth. Nelfinavir is an alternative agent that can be used, in particular if the mother is known to have developed resistance to AZT. Triple therapy is not usually indicated at birth, but may be initiated if there were an increasing viral load or a decreasing CD4 count. PCR (polymerase chain reaction) for HIV is usually performed within 48 hours, and repeated at 6 weeks. If both are negative therapy can be stopped and the baby followed up until an antibody-negative status is achieved. Babies should not be breast-fed, and should not receive BCG vaccination. Co-trimoxazole would usually be given from 6 weeks of age. There is no indication for immunoglobulin therapy.

12.12 C: To administer zoster immune globulin within 48 hours

Chickenpox is infectious from 24–48 hours before the rash appears until the final lesion has crusted. In an immunodeficient patient who is not immune to varicella zoster, there is a clear indication for zoster immune globulin. There would be a case for aciclovir to be given 7 days after exposure (minimum incubation time), but it is of little benefit until lesions develop. It may be necessary to suspend the programme of chemotherapy, but the most appropriate action is to give zoster immune globulin within 48 hours.

12.13 A: Interferon-α and ribavirin

A combination of interferon-α and ribavirin has been shown to be effective in chronic hepatitis C infection, and is given for 6–12 months. Treatment is usually initiated on the basis of changes in liver biopsy histology, and success is tracked by measuring viral loads. Interferon-α alone is less effective, and ribavirin used alone is ineffective. Lamivudine is used in hepatitis B infection. Interferon-γ is of benefit in chronic granulomatous disease and in treating atypical mycobacterial infection in patients with defects of the interleukin-12 / interferon-γ axis.

EMQ Answers

12.14 UK vaccination schedule

1. A: At birth

Hepatitis B (active) vaccination should be given shortly after birth if the mother is a carrier. Further doses are given at 1, 2 and 12 months. Passive immunisation with hepatitis-B-specific immunoglobulin should also be given at birth if the mother has active hepatitis or is hepatitis B envelope antigen (HBeAg)-positive (or is hepatitis B surface antigen [HBsAg]-positive and the e marker status is unknown). The two injections should not be given at the same site.

2. G: 12 months

A family history of inflammatory bowel disease should not alter the timing of MMR vaccination.

3.   C: 2 months

The current routine schedule (2009) for the UK is as follows:

Age	Vaccine
2 months	DPT, inactivated polio, HIB (5 in 1) Pneumococcal
3 months	DPT, inactivated polio, HIB MenC
4 months	DPT, inactivated polio, HIB Pneumococcal MenC
~12 months	HIB MenC
~13 months	MMR Pneumococcal
~3 years, 4 months (pre-school booster)	DPT, inactivated polio MMR
Girls aged 12–13 years	HPV
13–18 years	DT, inactivated polio

DPT, diphtheria/pertussis/tetanus; HIB, *Haemophilus influenzae* type B; HPV, human papillomavirus types 16 & 18; MenC, meningococcal meningitis type C; MMR, measles/mumps/rubella. The recently deployed 5-in-1 vaccine includes inactivated polio and HIB in the same injection as DTP.

12.15 Immune cells

1.   A: B cells

B cells are reduced (< 2%) or absent in X-linked agammaglobulinaemia. This disorder is also known as Bruton's disease. Failure to produce B cells causes loss of immunoglobulin production. Infants are initially protected by maternal IgG, but then present with recurrent pulmonary, middle-ear and sinus infections. Lifelong replacement therapy with immunoglobulin therapy is required.

2.   J: Dendritic cells

Dendritic cells are professional antigen-presenting cells and interact closely with T cells.

3   C: CD8 T cells

T cells expressing CD8 encode class I MHC restricted T-cell receptors and are capable of destroying virally infected cells.

13. Infectious diseases

Multiple True–False Questions

13.1 Which of the following are true of chickenpox?
- [ ] A the rash starts on the trunk and spreads outwards
- [ ] B household contacts are less severely affected than the index case
- [ ] C the rash is preceded by a viraemia
- [ ] D respiratory secretions are highly infectious
- [ ] E the rash is erythematous in nature

13.2 Immunocompromised children are at particular risk from the following infections:
- [ ] A rotavirus
- [ ] B *Pneumocystis jiroveci* pneumonia
- [ ] C cytomegalovirus
- [ ] D pneumococcal pneumonia
- [ ] E enterovirus

13.3 Which of the following statements about human immunodeficiency virus (HIV) infection in children are correct?
- [ ] A most babies are infected by horizontal transmission from their mothers
- [ ] B infected babies can present in the first 6 months of life with *Pneumocystis jiroveci* pneumonia
- [ ] C children requiring treatment for HIV should receive a two-drug regimen
- [ ] D serial viral loads and CD4 counts are used to monitor children with HIV
- [ ] E the life expectancy of children with HIV is thought to be around 20 years with treatment

13.4 The following can cause food-borne infections:
- [ ] A *Mycobacterium tuberculosis*
- [ ] B *Salmonella* spp.
- [ ] C *Staphylococcus aureus*
- [ ] D *Listeria monocytogenes*
- [ ] E *Clostridium tetani*

13.5   Cats are carriers of the following:

☐ A toxoplasmosis
☐ B psittacosis
☐ C echinococcosis
☐ D *Bartonella henselae*
☐ E leptospirosis

13.6   Measles is classically characterised by

☐ A a fine maculopapular rash starting behind the ears
☐ B Koplick spots on the face
☐ C convulsions
☐ D coryza
☐ E diarrhoea

13.7   Which of the following complications is a 12-year-old boy with orbital cellulitis at risk of developing?

☐ A meningitis
☐ B cavernous sinus thrombosis
☐ C cerebral abscess
☐ D cerebral artery embolus
☐ E epistaxis

13.8   A 1-year-old child presenting with which of the following conditions would need further investigation of their immune function?

☐ A herpes stomatitis
☐ B cytomegalovirus (CMV) pneumonitis
☐ C two previous admissions – one with meningitis, one with pneumonia
☐ D six viral upper respiratory infections in 1 year
☐ E an atypical mycobacterial cold abscess of the cervical node

Best of Five Questions

13.9 A 3-year-old girl with vertically acquired HIV has recently started antiretroviral therapy. Which of the following sets of investigations would be BEST to monitor efficacy of treatment?

☐ A   CD4 and CD8 counts
☐ B   Lymphocyte count and viral load
☐ C   HIV antibody and CD4 count
☐ D   HIV viral load and CD4 count
☐ E   Immunoglobulins

13.10 Which of the following diseases is NOT found in Britain?

☐ A   Toxoplasmosis
☐ B   Rabies
☐ C   Lyme disease
☐ D   Echinococcosis
☐ E   *Bartonella henselae* infection

13.11 Which of the following tests is the one ROUTINELY offered to mothers as part of antenatal care in the UK?

☐ A   toxoplasmosis
☐ B   HIV
☐ C   high vaginal swab for group B *Streptococcus*
☐ D   high vaginal swab for herpes simplex virus type 2
☐ E   cytomegalovirus

13.12 The following children have been exposed to a case of chickenpox. Which one does NOT require specific varicella zoster immunoglobulin?

☐ A   A child currently on chemotherapy
☐ B   A child who had a bone marrow transplant 1 month previously
☐ C   A child with a kidney transplant who is receiving immunosuppressive treatment
☐ D   A child who has had prednisolone 1 mg/kg for the past 6 weeks
☐ E   A child who had prednisolone 2 mg/kg for 3 days 1 week ago

13.13 An 11-year-old boy in the UK presents with a 10-day history of headache, sore throat, chest pain, and dry cough. His GP gave him a course of amoxicillin 4 days ago, but he is no better and is now coughing up yellow sputum and is wheezy. He also complains of abdominal pain and painful swollen knees. Which of the following organisms is MOST likely to be the cause of his illness?

- ☐ A *Streptococcus pneumoniae*
- ☐ B *Mycoplasma pneumoniae*
- ☐ C *Mycobacterium tuberculosis*
- ☐ D *Chlamydia trachomatis*
- ☐ E *Haemophilus influenzae*

Extended Matching Questions

13.14 Theme: Infections in the infant

A Enterovirus
B Group B *Streptococcus*
C Meningococcus
D Toxoplasmosis
E Cytomegalovirus
F *Pneumocystis jiroveci*
G Herpes simplex virus (HSV)
H *Haemophilus influenzae type B*
I Syphilis
J Adenovirus
K Rubella

For each of the following case scenarios select the most likely causative organism from the list above. Each option may be used once, more than once, or not at all.

- ☐ 1. A 2-month-old white boy presents in summer, febrile and in severe respiratory distress, with marked intercostal recession and tracheal tug. He has no audible crackles or wheeze on auscultation. His temperature is 37.8 °C, his pulse 70 beats/min, respiratory rate 70 breaths/min, and blood pressure 90/56 mmHg. He has an oxygen saturation of 76% in air. His arterial blood gas values are: pH 7.25, PO_2 6.9 kPa, PCO_2 4.3 kPa, base excess −9 mmol/L. Other laboratory values are: haemoglobin 9.2 g/dL (normal range [NR] 10.5–14 g/dL), white cell count (WCC) 12 × 10^9/L (NR 6–15 × 10^9/L), platelets 100 × 10^9/L (NR 150–450 × 10^9/L), neutrophils 9.5 × 10^9/L, lymphocytes 2.5 × 10⁹/L, eosinophils 0.3 × 10⁹/L, bilirubin 15 μmol/L (NR 1.7–26 μmol/L), aspartate aminotransferase (AST) 40 U/L (NR 10–45 U/L), serum sodium 136 mmol/L (NR 135–145 mmol/L), serum potassium 3.9 mmol/L (NR 3.5–5.6 mmol/L), serum urea 4.5 μmol/L (NR 2.5–6.6 mmol/L).

2. A 5-week-old baby presents with unusual posturing for the past 24 hours. He has been afebrile, feeding slightly less than usual, has a weak, high-pitched cry, and is irritable. He was born at term, by normal vaginal delivery, and was discharged at 24 hours. The pregnancy was normal and the mother well throughout. He is not jaundiced. He has a bulging fontanelle and is hypertonic. Laboratory results show: haemoglobin 11.2 g/dL, WCC 29.3 × 10⁹/L, neutrophils 60%, lymphocytes 28%, platelets 130 × 10⁹/L, erythrocyte sedimentation rate (ESR) 50 mm/h, C-reactive protein (CRP) 10 mg/dL, sodium 131 mmol/L, potassium 4.2 mmol/L, urea 4.9 mmol/L, creatinine 39 μmol/L, glucose 6.5 mmol/L; blood cultures negative; cerebrospinal fluid (CSF): protein 1.9 g/L, glucose 4.0 mmol/L, chloride normal; microscopy: red blood cells (RBC) 3 × 10¹²/L, WBC 350 × 10⁹/L, neutrophils 30%, lymphocytes 70%.

3. An 8-day-old baby presents with tachypnoea, poor feeding, and a capillary refill time of 4 seconds. She was born at term after a 3-day prolonged rupture of membranes. Examination revealed an enlarged liver, easy bruising and a rash. Initial investigations were as follows: haemoglobin 14 g/dL (NR 10.5–14 g/dL), WCC 8 × 10⁹/L (NR 6–15 × 10⁹/L), urea 8 mmol/L (NR 2.5–6.6 mmol/L), creatinine 68 μmol/L (NR 20–80 μmol/L), pH 7.28 (NR 7.32–7.37), bicarbonate 19 mmol/L, PCO₂ 4.0 kPa; base excess –9 mmol/L, alanine aminotransferase (ALT) 787 U/L (NR 10–40 U/L), prothrombin time (PT) grossly abnormal, activated partial thromboplastin time (APPT) grossly abnormal, CRP 4 mg/dL (NR < 5 mg/dL), O₂ saturations in air 97%.

13.15 Theme: Imported infectious diseases

A Giardia
B Yellow fever
C Typhoid
D Malaria
E Rocky Mountain spotted fever
F Tetanus
G Ehrlichiosis
H Ebola
I Dengue fever
J Babesiosis

For each of the following case scenarios, select the most likely diagnosis from the list above. Each option may be used once, more than once, or not at all.

☐ 1. A 4-year-old girl, returned from holiday in India, presents with a 4-week history of swinging fevers, diarrhoea, general malaise and a rash. Her temperature is 38 °C, pulse 80 beats/min, respiratory rate 15 breaths/min, and blood pressure (BP) 100/60 mmHg. Laboratory investigations reveal: haemoglobin 10 g/dL (NR 10.5–14 g/dL), WCC 6 × 10⁹/L (NR 6–15 × 10⁹/L), platelets 80 × 10⁹/L, neutrophils 2.0 × 10⁹/L, lymphocytes 2.5 × 10⁹/L, eosinophils 0.3 × 10⁹/L (NR 150–400 × 10⁹/L), bilirubin 20 μmol/L (NR 1.7–26 μmol/L), aspartate aminotransferase (AST) 80 U/L (NR 10–45 U/L), serum sodium 129 mmol/L (NR 135–145 mmol/L), serum potassium 3.7 mmol/L (NR 3.5–5.6 mmol/L), serum urea 6.5 mmol/L (2.5–6.6 mmol/L).

☐ 2. A 6-year-old boy, recently returned from the USA, presents with a 3-day history of severe headache, abdominal pain, nausea and vomiting, photophobia with marked neck stiffness, a gallop rhythm, a soft, tender abdomen with a palpable liver edge, and a petechial rash over the palms and soles of his feet, ankles, wrists, legs, and trunk. His temperature is 39.7 °C, pulse 170 beats/min, BP 95/50 mmHg; the capillary refill time is 3 s. Full blood count reveals: haemoglobin 9.2 g/dL, WCC 3.1 × 10⁹/L, neutrophils 1.2 × 10⁹/L, lymphocytes 0.8 × 10⁹/L, platelets 40 × 10⁹/L. Other laboratory results are: sodium 123 mmol/L (NR 135–145 mmol/L), potassium 3.0 mmol/L (NR 3.5–5.6 mmol/L), urea 4 mmol/L (NR 2.5–6.6 mmol/L), creatinine 23 μmol/L, AST 230 U/L (NR 10–45 U/L), bilirubin 5 μmol/L (NR 1.7–26 μmol/L), international normalised ratio (INR) 1.5, APTT 22 s, PT 13 s.

☐ 3. A 5-year-old who returned from Ghana the previous week presents
        with a 2-week history of spiking fevers, vomiting, and a cough. His
        temperature is 39 °C, pulse is 120 beats/min, respiratory rate
        20 breaths/min, BP 105/58 mmHg. Blood analysis reveals:
        haemoglobin 7.6 g/dL (NR 10.5–14 g/dL), WCC 10 × 10⁹/L
        (NR 6–15 × 10⁹/L), platelets 80 × 10⁹/L (NR 150–450 × 10⁹/L),
        neutrophils 4.0 × 10⁹/L, lymphocytes 4.5 × 10⁹/L, eosinophils
        0.2 × 10⁹/L, bilirubin 45 μmol/L (NR 1.7–26 μmol/L), AST 39 U/L
        (NR 10–45 U/L), serum sodium 131 mmol/L (NR 135–145 mmol/L),
        serum potassium 4.2 mmol/L (NR 3.5–5.6 mmol/L), serum urea
        7.5 mmol/L (NR 2.5–6.6 mmol/L).

MT–F Answers

13.1 Chickenpox: A C D

The rash of chickenpox is vesicular and centripetal. It starts on the trunk and spreads outwards. The last lesions to occur are those on the hands and feet. The rash is preceded by a viraemia and respiratory symptoms, with high viral loads in respiratory secretions. This is a particularly infectious period. Because of the close proximity and longer periods of contact, household contacts tend to become infected with higher viral loads than the index cases, and disease in these patients is more severe.

13.2 Infections from which immunocompromised children are at particular risk: B C

Immunocompromised children are at risk of infection with *Pneumocystis jiroveci* (formerly known as *Pneumocystis carinii*) and cytomegalovirus, both of which can cause severe pneumonitis. Rotavirus, *Pneumococcus* and enteroviruses are all pathogens that cause disease in immunocompetent patients in addition to the immunocompromised.

13.3 HIV infection in children: B D

Most babies are infected by vertical transmission from an HIV-positive mother. Approximately two-thirds of infections occur intrapartum (at delivery), and one third occur antenatally. Breast feeding doubles the transmission rate and is not recommended in the developed world. Mother-to-child transmission can be reduced from approximately 30% to less than 1% with the following measures:

- antiretroviral therapy (ART) given to the mother in pregnancy to decrease viral load to < 50 copies/mL
- ART given to the baby for the first 4–6 weeks of life
- delivery by lower-segment caesarean section (LSCS), preventing prolonged rupture of membranes
- avoidance of breast-feeding.

Babies should be diagnosed by polymerase chain reaction (PCR) if under 18 months of age, as maternal antibody can persist this long and so give false-positive results. It is important to give antiretroviral therapy to the infant as soon as possible after birth. Standard treatment for children requiring treatment is triple therapy with antiretroviral agents. Infected children are monitored using viral loads and CD4 counts to determine when treatment is required and to monitor it once it has been started. Average life expectancy is around 40 years.

13.4 Organisms causing food-borne infections: B C D

Salmonella spp. and *Staphylococcus aureus* are common causes of food poisoning. *Listeria monocytogenes* causes sporadic outbreaks of food poisoning, and asymptomatic carriage in pregnant women can lead to neonatal sepsis. *Mycobacterium tuberculosis* is not a cause of food poisoning, although bovine mycobacterial strains can cause intestinal tuberculosis, which is very rare. *Clostridium tetani* is widespread in soil and causes neurological disease in unvaccinated patients when introduced through wound sites. It is another strain of *Clostridium*, *C. botulinum*, which causes severe and devastating toxin-mediated food poisoning.

13.5 Diseases carried by cats: A D

Toxoplasmosis and *Bartonella henselae* (the causative organism of cat-scratch disease) are both carried by cats. Psittacosis is carried by birds, and *Echinococcus* is found in dogs, both wild and domestic. *Leptospira* is carried by rats.

13.6 Features of measles: A D

Measles characteristically presents with a prodromal illness, which includes coryzal symptoms (runny nose), non-purulent conjunctivitis and a brassy cough, followed by a rash. Koplik spots appear as grey-white lesions on the buccal mucosa. The typical rash is maculopapular, starting behind the ears, spreading to the face and down the trunk. The lesions tend to coalesce and fade to a dusky colour. Children often have a sore mouth, but diarrhoea is not common. Convulsions are not a characteristic feature of measles, and if they occur they are invariably triggered by the fever, or reflect encephalitis.

13.7 Orbital cellulitis: A B C

There are many serious potential complications from orbital cellulitis. These include involvement of the optic nerve, leading to loss of vision, and intracranial extension of infection, leading to meningitis and intracranial abscesses. Cavernous sinus thrombosis is another well-recognised complication, because the venous drainage around the orbit and face is back into the cavernous sinus. Finally, it is always worth imaging the sinuses because orbital cellulitis is often associated with underlying sinusitis.

13.8   Investigation of immune function: B C

Cytomegalovirus (CMV) pneumonitis is unusual in children with normal immune function, but children with T-cell dysfunction such as HIV or SCID can present with it. Any child with two serious bacterial infections, such as meningitis and pneumonia, needs investigation of their immune system. The occurrence of more than 10–15 upper respiratory tract infections in a year may indicate a minor immunodeficiency. Herpes stomatitis and atypical mycobacterial skin infections do not require further investigation if they are the only infections a child has had.

Best of Five Answers

13.9   D: HIV viral load and CD4 count

Antiretroviral treatment is monitored by looking at the CD4 count and the HIV viral load. HIV antibodies may be used in diagnosing HIV infection, although children younger than 18 months may still have maternally acquired HIV antibodies. High immunoglobulin levels occur in HIV-infected children but are non-specific. Viral load is **not** the same as HIV antigen, as the latter is qualitative, detecting the presence or absence of antigen; viral load is quantitative, looking at the amount of HIV virus in the blood, and is measured in copies/mL. Fewer than 50 copies/mL is deemed 'undetectable' and is a sign that the HIV virus is being successfully suppressed by medication (not eradicated, as antiretroviral therapy is only able to suppress viral replication).

13.10 B: Rabies

Rabies is the only one of these diseases that is not found in Britain. Lyme disease is endemic in parts of the Lake District, and is found in deer elsewhere in the country. *Echinococcus* is found in rural regions, mainly in sheep-farming areas. Both toxoplasmosis and *Bartonella henselae* are carried by cats, with humans being accidental hosts.

13.11 B: HIV

HIV testing is routinely offered to pregnant women as part of their routine antenatal care. It is provided on an 'opt-out' basis – ie, those who don't want to be HIV tested need specifically to refuse the test. Toxoplasmosis and cytomegalovirus, although both causing congenital infection, are rare, and therefore it is not cost-effective to screen for them as part of routine antenatal care. High vaginal swabs are performed on women deemed at risk for these diseases only.

13.12 E: A child who had prednisolone 2 mg/kg for 3 days 1 week ago

Note that this means that a child receiving the standard 3-day course of steroids for an acute exacerbation of asthma would not require varicella zoster immunoglobulin after exposure to chickenpox. All the other children described are immunocompromised to some degree, and so would require it.

13.13 B: *Mycoplasma pneumoniae*

This is a typical description of *Mycoplasma pneumoniae* infection. The history is too short for tuberculosis. *Streptococcus* and *Haemophilus* do not cause the extrapulmonary symptoms, and *Chlamydia* causes a chest infection in babies aged 4–6 weeks.

EMQ Answers

13.14 Infections in the infant

1. F: *Pneumocystis jiroveci*

This is a classic presentation of *Pneumocystis jiroveci* pneumonia (PCP). Immunocompromised children present in the first 6 months of life, with a peak at 2–3 months of age. They have severe respiratory compromise, little to hear on auscultation, and marked hypoxia. Cytomegalovirus (CMV) is the second most likely option, and in the absence of PCP, can cause this clinical picture in the immunocompromised host.

2. A: Enterovirus

This baby has meningitis. The protein (only slightly raised for this age group), normal chloride and CSF glucose, with a white cell count that is raised (but not in the thousands), with a predominant lymphocytosis, makes a viral meningitis the most likely cause. Enterovirus is the most common cause of viral meningitis. HSV needs to be considered, but this patient is just outside the neonatal age range, the CSF red cell count is low, and he has no other stigmata of HSV, making this less likely to be the causative organism. Again, considering the age of the baby, group B *Streptococcus* and *Haemophilus influenzae* need to be considered, but he is just beyond the at-risk age for the first, and, although he has not yet been immunised against the latter, its incidence in the community has decreased drastically as a result of 'herd immunity'.

3. G: Herpes simplex virus

As often is the case in clinical practice, the neonate presents with non-specific signs and symptoms of sepsis. In this case the baby is a little older, has an enlarged liver, grossly abnormal liver function tests and clotting. The white blood cell count and CRP are normal, suggesting a non-bacterial cause; however, the prolonged rupture of membranes gives a clue to an infective cause. The rash is actually vesicular, and the baby has disseminated herpes simplex virus (HSV) infection. This classically presents around this time, usually in the offspring of a mother who has acquired HSV late in the third trimester (the infection is often an asymptomatic in the mother). Approximately 85% of neonatal HSV infections are acquired at delivery, 5% prenatally, and 10% postnatally (eg from cold sores, herpetic whitlow). Without early treatment with intravenous aciclovir, the mortality is extremely high. Other diagnoses, in order of likelihood, are as follows: metabolic disease, overwhelming bacterial sepsis (still the most common neonatal diagnosis, even if not the most likely in this case), enterovirus infection, syphilis, and other congenital infections. Congenital heart disease may give rise to poor feeding and enlarged liver, but not grossly abnormal liver function tests or deranged clotting.

13.15 Imported infectious diseases

1. C: Typhoid

Typhoid typically presents with a relative bradycardia in association with the pyrexia. Often the eosinophil and platelet counts are low. AST can be raised and hyponatraemia is common. With this long history, HIV has to be considered. Malaria must also be excluded.

2. E: Rocky Mountain spotted fever

There are a number of tick-borne infectious diseases that occur in North America. Rocky Mountain spotted fever is a rickettsial disease carried by ticks in the area of the Rocky Mountains, and peaks in the summer. It is acute, can be fatal, and presents classically, as in this child, with severe headache, a fine petechial rash, and derangement of liver functions and electrolytes. In this country, meningococcal disease is the obvious differential diagnosis. However, although sporadic cases occur in the summer, it peaks in the winter season. Ehrlichiosis would be another choice on this list. It also occurs in the USA, tends to be found more commonly in the south-west of the country, and is often known as 'spotless', as the disease presentation is very similar, but without the rash. Treatment of Rocky Mountain spotted fever is with either chloramphenicol or doxycycline, so recognition and diagnosis are important, as neither of these are antibiotics used in the normal course of events in septic children here in the UK.

3.   D: Malaria

A child with malaria can present acutely unwell, often with a fever and cough. Severe diarrhoea is rare. They are often anaemic, with a raised bilirubin but normal liver function tests. Tuberculosis is the second possibility – although less likely, as the history is relatively short. Typhoid is a great mimic of other diseases, and is the third choice.

14. Metabolic Medicine

Multiple True–False Questions

14.1 Dietary protein restriction is a feature of the management of
- [ ] A phenylketonuria (PKU)
- [ ] B non-ketotic hyperglycinaemia (NKH)
- [ ] C glucose transporter 1 (GLUT 1) deficiency
- [ ] D argininosuccinic aciduria
- [ ] E methylmalonic acidaemia

14.2 An increased urinary methylmalonate concentration in a neonatal sample may be seen in
- [ ] A classic homocystinuria
- [ ] B propionic acidaemia
- [ ] C cobalamin C deficiency
- [ ] D the infant of a vegetarian mother
- [ ] E folate deficiency

14.3 Gluconeogenesis
- [ ] A occurs in the cytosol
- [ ] B converts glycogen to glucose
- [ ] C is activated by insulin
- [ ] D is inhibited by alcohol
- [ ] E if defective, presents with hypoketotic hypoglycaemia

14.4 Which of the following is true of glutaric aciduria type 1?
- [ ] A microcephaly is a feature
- [ ] B may be misdiagnosed as non-accidental injury
- [ ] C presents at birth
- [ ] D IQ is normal
- [ ] E inheritance is autosomal recessive

14.5 Recognised features of cystinuria include:
- [ ] A photophobia
- [ ] B growth faltering
- [ ] C renal calculi
- [ ] D diabetes mellitus
- [ ] E rickets

14.6 **Which of the following statements about phenylketonuria (PKU) are true?**

☐ A   breast-feeding is contraindicated in the newborn infant with phenylketonuria

☐ B   the diet is phenylalanine-free

☐ C   the concentration of brain phenylalanine directly correlates with that in the plasma

☐ D   'diet' drinks (with artificial sweeteners) improve phenylalanine control

☐ E   phenylalanine is teratogenic

Best of Five Questions

14.7 **A 3-month-old infant was referred for investigation for poor weight gain. On examination, a 2-cm hepatomegaly was noted, and the presence of immature cataracts bilaterally. Investigations revealed: pH 7.32, standard bicarbonate 15.8 mmol/L, base excess −8 mmol/L, sodium 134 mmol/L, potassium 3.4 mmol/L, chloride 106 mmol/L, lactate 1.9 mmol/L. What is the MOST likely cause of the acid–base disturbance?**

☐ A   Renal tubular acidosis

☐ B   Organic acidaemia

☐ C   Lactic acidosis

☐ D   Ketolysis defect

☐ E   Urea cycle defect

14.8 **A 2-month-old male infant presents with cough and poor feeding. The infant is floppy and has a 3-cm palpable liver below the costal margin. A chest X-ray reveals cardiomegaly, confirmed on echocardiography, demonstrating hypertrophic cardiomyopathy. Further investigations include an electrocardiogram (ECG) that reveals giant QRS complexes, and examination of a blood film that confirms the presence of vacuolated lymphocytes. The MOST likely diagnosis is which of the following?**

☐ A   Mitochondrial cardiomyopathy

☐ B   Fat oxidation defect

☐ C   Barth syndrome

☐ D   Pompe syndrome

☐ E   Hurler syndrome

14.9 The third child of unrelated parents required ventilation for increasing apnoeas on the second day of life. The pregnancy had been uneventful and the mother reported that the baby was very active in utero, with no decrease in fetal movements. Shortly after delivery, the infant was noted to be floppy, with frequent hiccoughs. Septic screen was negative and cerebral ultrasound was reported as normal. Ammonia and lactate are normal. What is the next KEY investigation?

☐ A Plasma amino acids
☐ B Biotinidase assay
☐ C Urinary sulphite dipstick
☐ D Trial of pyridoxine
☐ E Urinary organic acids

14.10 A 5-year-old boy was found to have a poor cortisol response when hypoglycaemic. On the basis of the results of further investigations shown below, what is the MOST likely diagnosis?

Synacthen test			
Time (min)	0	30	60
Cortisol (nmol/l)	102	93	87
Very-long-chain fatty acids			
C24 / C22 ratio	1.53	(NR < 0.96)	
C26 / C22 ratio	0.057	(NR < 0.022)	
NR, normal range.			

☐ A MCAD deficiency
☐ B Zellweger syndrome
☐ C Addison's disease
☐ D Adrenoleukodystrophy
☐ E Glutaric aciduria type 1

14.11 A 10-month-old girl presented with pneumonia. She was noted to have marked hepatomegaly. Before she starting receiving intravenous fluids, the laboratory glucose was 2.1 mmol/L. Further investigations revealed: lactate 6.1 mmol/L (normal range [NR] < 2.0 mmol/L), triglycerides 17 mmol/L (NR < 2.3 mmol/L), urate 3.6 mmol/L (NR < 0.47 mmol/L). The MOST likely diagnosis is which of the following?

☐ A Phosphofructokinase deficiency (glycogen storage disorder [GSD] V)
☐ B Glucose-6-phosphatase deficiency (GSD I)
☐ C Branching enzyme deficiency (GSD IV)
☐ D Debrancher enzyme deficiency (GSD III)
☐ E Myophosphorylase deficiency (GSD VII)

14.12 A 48-hour-old infant on the postnatal ward is noted to be tachypnoeic, sleepy, and feeding poorly. Blood-gas analysis shows: pH 7.48, PaO_2 12.3 kPa, $PaCO_2$ 3.6 kPa, standard bicarbonate 20.0 mmol/L; base excess 1.6 mmol/L. What is the NEXT key investigation?

☐ A Ammonia
☐ B Lactate
☐ C Chest X-ray
☐ D Amino acids
☐ E Blood culture

14.13 A 12-month-old girl was referred for investigation for developmental regression, having lost the ability to sit unsupported. Fundus examination revealed a cherry-red spot. There were no audible murmurs, and the abdomen was soft with no palpable organomegaly. What is the MOST likely diagnosis?

☐ A Fabry's disease
☐ B Sandhoff's disease
☐ C Niemann–Pick type C
☐ D Gaucher's disease
☐ E Tay–Sachs disease

Extended Matching Questions

14.14 Theme: Interpretation of amino acids

A   Phenylketonuria
B   Tyrosinaemia
C   3-Phosphoglycerine dehydrogenase deficiency
D   Non-ketotic hyperglycinaemia
E   Ornithine transcarbamylase deficiency
F   Maple syrup urine disease
G   Propionic acidaemia
H   Leigh syndrome
I   Hyperinsulinism

For each of the following amino acid results, select from the list above the most likely diagnosis. Each option may be used once, more than once, or not at all.

☐   1.

Amino acid	Value (μmol/L)	Normal range (μmol/L)
Serine	129	51–231
Glutamine	453	307–768
Glycine	222	81–303
Leucine	1137	50–264
Isoleucine	457	26–159
Valine	826	96–566
Arginine	102	26–180
Phenylalanine	75	34–110
Tyrosine	63	26–154

☐ 2.

Amino acid	Value (μmol/L)	Normal range (μmol/L)
Serine	124	51–231
Glutamine	4188	307–768
Glycine	301	81–303
Leucine	231	50–264
Isoleucine	74	26–159
Valine	320	96–566
Arginine	17	26–180
Phenylalanine	59	34–110
Tyrosine	276	26–154

☐ 3.

Amino acid	Value (μmol/L)	Normal range (μmol/L)
Serine	186	51–231
Glutamine	324	307–768
Glycine	316	81–303
Leucine	121	50–264
Isoleucine	71	26–159
Valine	193	96–566
Arginine	36	26–180
Phenylalanine	1419	34–110
Tyrosine	52	26–154

14.15 Theme: Investigations of inborn errors

A Very-long-chain fatty acids
B Urinary sulphite dipstick
C Urinary amino acids
D Plasma amino acids
E Organic acids
F Acyl carnitines
G Urinary urate
H Plasma urate
I Ammonia
J 7-Dehydrocholesterol

For each of the following inborn errors, select the most appropriate initial investigation from the list above. Each option may be used once, more than once, or not at all.

☐ 1. Zellweger syndrome.
☐ 2. Smith–Lemli–Opitz syndrome.
☐ 3. Lesch–Nyhan syndrome.

MT–F Answers

14.1   Dietary protein restriction: A C D E

Protein restriction is a common strategy for many aminoacidopathies, urea cycle defects, and organic acidaemias. In amino acid disorders, general protein restriction helps bring down the raised amino acid in question – eg phenylalanine in PKU, tyrosine in tyrosinaemia. An amino acid supplement containing all the other amino acids that would be deficient as a result of the dietary restriction is then given. Reducing protein in urea cycle defects decreases the nitrogen load on the urea cycle, helping control ammonia levels, eg in argininosuccinic aciduria. Similarly, protein restriction in organic acidaemias reduces organic acid build-up, as fewer amino acids are catabolised. GLUT 1 deficiency is managed with a ketogenic diet, to provide an alternative fuel for the brain, to combat the block in transfer of glucose across the blood–brain barrier. It is usually prescribed as a ratio of fat to carbohydrate and protein (eg 3:1 or 4:1) and therefore protein is restricted and the diet is quite limited. It is not the same as an Atkins diet, which is a lot more palatable and varied because only carbohydrate is restricted. Protein restriction in NKH is ineffective in controlling seizures, and therefore is not used.

14.2   Neonatal increase in methylmalonate: C D

Increased methylmalonate is a not infrequent finding in neonates who have organic acid analysis as part of their investigation. Pathological causes include methylmalonic aciduria and vitamin B_{12} deficiency. The latter may reflect poor maternal stores, as seen in vegetarians and mothers with pernicious anaemias (although this may not yet have been diagnosed). Investigation therefore includes vitamin B_{12} levels in both the neonate and mother, along with organic acids in the mother. Vitamin B_{12} deficiency also results from disorders of B_{12} metabolism, cobalamin C defects being the most common. Key findings include low B_{12}, and increased methylmalonate and homocysteine. Some neonates have minimally elevated levels of methylmalonate that improve with age, probably related to improving dietary intake of B_{12}. The increase usually resolves with a short course of B_{12}, without the infant showing improvement in the symptoms that were being investigated.

14.3   Gluconeogenesis: A D

Gluconeogenesis is the de-novo synthesis of glucose from non-carbohydrate sources such as amino acids, lactate and glycerol. It occurs within the cytosol, apart from the first step, which occurs in the mitochondria. It is activated by glucagon and suppressed by insulin. Alcohol inhibits gluconeogenesis, and so should not be taken in excess in patients at risk of hypoglycaemia, eg those with defects of fat oxidation. Defects of gluconeogenesis present with fasting hypoglycaemia and lactic acidosis, because of the failure to recycle lactate to glucose. Ketosis is a feature.

14.4   Glutaric aciduria type 1: B D E

Glutaric aciduria type 1 is an autosomal recessive condition usually presenting towards the end of the first year of life with metabolic decompensation precipitated, like many other inborn errors, by intercurrent illness. Before this, the only clue may be macrocephaly, which makes the children more vulnerable to subdural bleeds from the stretched bridging veins. This combination of subdural bleeds and encephalopathy has led to misdiagnosis of non-accidental injury. Urinary organic acid analysis should therefore be undertaken in such children to exclude an inappropriate diagnosis. Basal ganglia damage post-decompensation is common, with resultant chorea and dystonia. IQ is normal. Extended newborn screening is undertaken in some countries with the aim that decompensation can be avoided by dietary manipulation and aggressive management of intercurrent infections.

14.5   Cystinuria: C

Cystinuria is a transport defect resulting in the excessive loss of COAL (cystine, ornithine, arginine and lysine) in the urine. The only clinical consequence is the formation of renal stones. All the listed features are seen in cystinosis. This is a lysosomal defect; excess cystine is stored, with adverse effects on kidneys, liver, thyroid, pancreas and brain.

14.6   Phenylketonuria (PKU): E

PKU results from a block in phenylalanine metabolism, resulting in increased phenylalanine levels and neurological impairment. It is managed with a phenylalanine-restricted diet. Phenylalanine is an essential amino acid and therefore cannot be totally removed from the diet. In the neonate it can be given as formula or breast milk. The level of phenylalanine in the brain cannot be predicted from the plasma concentration, which explains why some patients have good outcomes despite poor control, and vice versa. A reduction in transport across the blood–brain barrier is protective. 'Diet' drinks are contraindicated because aspartame contains phenylalanine, so the full-sugar varieties are preferred. Phenylalanine is teratogenic, and therefore even though the chance of a PKU mother having a PKU-affected child is only 1 in 100, the fetus can still be damaged by maternal PKU. The condition must be managed very carefully in pregnancy, by more frequent blood monitoring and stricter control of phenylalanine concentrations.

Best of Five Answers

14.7   A: Renal tubular acidosis

The investigations reveal a metabolic acidosis with a normal anion gap: sodium + potassium – (chloride + bicarbonate). Normal range is 10–18 mmol/L. This suggests bicarbonate loss rather than an excess of acid. The most likely causes would therefore be renal or gut loss of bicarbonate. The hepatomegaly and cataracts would be suggestive of galactosaemia. Some patients do not present in the newborn period, but might present later with the renal effects of galactosaemia, often with rickets secondary to the phosphate leak resulting from the renal Fanconi syndrome.

14.8   D: Pompe syndrome

Mitochondrial disorders, fat oxidation defects, and Pompe syndrome (glycogen storage disorder type II) are recognised causes of hypertrophic cardiomyopathy. Here, however, the presence of vacuolated lymphocytes indicating storage material confirms Pompe syndrome as the most likely cause. Presentation is usually within the first months of life, with hypotonia, weakness, hyporeflexia, and a large tongue. Creatine kinase is increased, but may be normal. The ECG may need to be recorded on half voltage so that the giant QRS complexes caused by gross ventricular hypertrophy can be accommodated on the page. Enzyme replacement therapy is now licensed for this disorder. Without treatment, most affected infants die in the first year of life. Barth syndrome is an X-linked cardiomyopathy, but presents with a dilated cardiomyopathy. Heart involvement in Hurler syndrome is usually with valve involvement in the second decade of life or later.

14.9   A: Plasma amino acids

The clinical presentation is very suggestive of non-ketotic hyperglycinaemia, and therefore elevation of glycine is a key diagnostic clue, with further confirmation gained from a concurrent cerebrospinal fluid to plasma ratio. Glycine is a neurotransmitter with central excitatory effects producing seizures, with peripheral inhibitory effects causing hypotonia. On direct questioning, mothers often report very active fetuses, which may correspond to in-utero seizures.

14.10 D: Adrenoleukodystrophy

The Synacthen test shows a flat response, with no increase in cortisol. The VLCFAs are increased, consistent with X-linked adrenoleukodystrophy (X-ALD). Forty per cent of boys with isolated adrenal insufficiency will have X-ALD. It is therefore essential to screen such patients for VLCFAs, to ensure the diagnosis is made a soon as possible. It is important to remember that adrenal involvement may precede brain involvement or be the only symptom.

14.11 B: Glucose-6-phosphatase deficiency (GSD I)

The options presented are all glycogen storage disorders (GSDs). Hypoglycaemia is not a feature of the muscle GSDs V (phosphofructokinase) and VII (myophosphorylase); later onset of muscle fatigue and myalgia is their usual presentation. Branching enzyme deficiency (GSD IV) produces long glycogen chains that act like amylopectin to produce cirrhosis and, ultimately, liver failure. Hypoglycaemia is a feature of the liver GSDs: GSD I (a or b), GSD III, GSD VI and GSD IX, although it is usually mild (or absent) in the last two conditions. Here, the results of the investigations identify glucose-6-phosphatase deficiency as the cause. The biochemical signature of GSD I is hypoglycaemia, with increased lactate, urate, and triglycerides. Hypoglycaemia occurs once the exogenous sources of glucose are exhausted as glycogenolysis and gluconeogenesis are blocked. Presentation may be delayed by many months as long as regular and frequent feeds are taken (eg prop-feeding or demand feeding overnight). Breakdown of glycogen to pyruvate is intact, however, and lactate is therefore produced as a secondary fuel for the brain. Conversion of lactate and pyruvate to fatty acids and cholesterol results in hyperlipidaemia. Uric acid production from glucose-6-phosphate is increased.

14.12 A: Ammonia

The finding of a respiratory alkalosis in a sick neonate is unusual, and is not consistent with acidosis or a primary lung pathology causing the tachypnoea. Ammonia is a respiratory stimulant that acts directly on the brainstem, and should be measured in any child with encephalopathy and a respiratory alkalosis.

14.13 E: Tay–Sachs disease

A cherry-red spot is seen in Niemann–Pick type C, Tay–Sachs disease, and Sandhoff's disease, all of which can present with developmental delay and regression. Tay–Sachs disease is not associated with organomegaly, unlike Niemann–Pick type C and Sandhoff's disease. Hyperacusis may be noted as being startled by sound, from an early age.

EMQ Answers

14.14 Interpretation of amino acids

1. F: Maple syrup urine disease (raised leucine, isoleucine, and valine)

The branched-chain amino acids, leucine, isoleucine and valine, share a common enzyme at the start of their catabolic pathway. Deficiency of the branched-chain oxo acid dehydrogenase therefore results in increases in all three amino acids, and is the basis for maple syrup urine disease. The condition gets its name from the sweet smell associated with the urine. The opposite is seen in hyperinsulinism, with suppression of the branched-chain amino acids as a result of the anabolic effects of insulin.

2. E: Ornithine transcarbamylase deficiency (raised glutamine, low arginine)

This amino acid profile suggests a defect of the urea cycle. Ammonia is 'mopped up' by glutamate with a resultant increase in glutamine, which is then transported to the liver for conversion to urea. Local build-up of glutamine in the brain may contribute to the encephalopathy by causing cerebral oedema as a result of its osmotic effect. Arginine is a non-essential amino acid that is made in the urea cycle, and therefore in these conditions is often low because of the block in the cycle. The exception is arginase deficiency, which has a diagnostically high level due to the failure to break down arginine.

3. A: Phenylketonuria (raised phenylalanine)

This is the basis of the newborn screening test for PKU. Phenylalanine hydroxylase converts phenylalanine to tyrosine, and therefore the ratio of phenylalanine to tyrosine is increased. Classic PKU is defined as a phenylalanine level greater than 1000 μmol/L.

14.15 Investigations of inborn errors

1. A: Very-long-chain fatty acids

Zellweger syndrome is a disorder of peroxisomal biogenesis. Increased concentrations of very-long-chain fatty acids (VLCFAs) are indicative of peroxisomal disorders, because very-long-chain fat oxidation occurs within peroxisomes.

2. J: 7-Dehydrocholesterol

Smith–Lemli–Opitz syndrome results from a block in the final step in cholesterol synthesis, with subsequent build-up of its immediate precursor, 7-dehydrocholesterol. It is the most common defect of sterol biosynthesis. Absolute cholesterol will be low, but may be missed with standard lipid analyses, as these often measure all the cholesterol species collectively. The condition is associated with dysmorphology, syndactyly of 2nd and 3rd toes, mental retardation, genital anomalies, renal anomalies and growth faltering.

3. G: Urinary urate

Lesch–Nyhan syndrome is a disorder of purine metabolism. Urate is grossly increased as a result of the block in purine salvage, resulting in increased purine synthesis. However, renal clearance in children is very high, and therefore the plasma concentration may be at the upper part of the normal range, whereas the urinary concentration will still be elevated. Urate measurement is a key initial investigation in purine disorders, but should be measured in urine as well as plasma, to avoid missing the diagnosis.

15. Neonatology

Multiple True–False Questions

15.1 **The following are true regarding group B *Streptococcus* (GBS) infection:**

☐ A approximately 1% of babies of colonised mothers become infected
☐ B it is a Gram-positive coccus
☐ C approximately 50% of mothers are colonised with GBS
☐ D it is a sexually transmitted disease
☐ E cefotaxime is the antibiotic of choice

15.2 **A male, term baby is noted to be pale at birth. He is otherwise well and haemoglobin is found to be 7.1 g/dL. The following are possible causes of this presentation:**

☐ A α-thalassaemia
☐ B β-thalassaemia
☐ C sickle cell disease
☐ D glucose-6-phosphate dehydrogenase (G6PD) deficiency
☐ E chronic feto-maternal transfusion

15.3 **Which of the following statements about perinatal mortality are true?**

☐ A stillbirth is defined as an in-utero death occurring after 18 weeks' gestation
☐ B the perinatal mortality rate is defined as stillbirths and deaths within 6 days of birth per 1000 live- and stillbirths
☐ C the perinatal mortality rate in England and Wales is approximately 15 per 1000
☐ D the neonatal mortality rate includes babies born at less than 24 weeks' gestation if they are live-born
☐ E the most common cause of neonatal death in the UK is congenital anomaly

15.4 The following circulatory changes occur around the time of birth in term babies:

- ☐ A closure of the ductus venosus
- ☐ B decreased breakdown of prostaglandin E$_2$ (PGE$_2$)
- ☐ C decreased left atrial pressure
- ☐ D decreased right atrial pressure
- ☐ E decreased pulmonary vascular resistance facilitated by nitric oxide

15.5 Which of the following statements are true concerning weight, fluids and skin?

- ☐ A the percentage of body weight due to extracellular fluid increases with gestation
- ☐ B normal weight loss after birth is due to extracellular fluid losses
- ☐ C pre-term babies have a lower surface area to weight ratio than term babies
- ☐ D pre-term babies have increased transepidermal water loss as a result of excess sweating
- ☐ E skin maturation in pre-term babies is accelerated by antenatal steroids

15.6 The following are recognised features of fetal alcohol syndrome:

- ☐ A macrocephaly
- ☐ B congenital heart disease
- ☐ C pre- and postnatal growth failure
- ☐ D neural tube defects
- ☐ E prune belly

Best of Five Questions

15.7 A term, female baby presents with seizures on the third day of life. On examination she is found to have weak femoral pulses and a small cleft palate. The MOST likely underlying diagnosis is:

- ☐ A Turner syndrome
- ☐ B Fetal alcohol syndrome
- ☐ C Trisomy 13
- ☐ D DiGeorge syndrome
- ☐ E Goldenhar syndrome

15.8 A baby was born at 38 weeks' gestation by caesarean section because of fetal distress. Labour was induced because of concerns regarding fetal growth. Routine maternal serological tests were normal on antenatal booking. Birth weight was 2.25 kg. There is hepatosplenomegaly and a purpuric rash. The platelet count is found to be 26 × 10^9/L. X-rays of the long bones show osteitic changes at the epiphyses. A cranial ultrasound scan is normal. The MOST likely diagnosis is congenital infection due to:

☐ A Rubella
☐ B Cytomegalovirus (CMV)
☐ C Toxoplasmosis
☐ D Human immunodeficiency virus (HIV)
☐ E Syphilis

15.9 A term baby has persistent hypoglycaemia in spite of receiving intravenous dextrose at 6–8 mg/kg per min. The MOST important investigation to request next is:

☐ A Check urine for presence of ketones
☐ B Urine organic acids
☐ C Blood insulin and C-peptide levels
☐ D Full blood count
☐ E Blood cortisol level

15.10 A term baby presented with severe respiratory failure, which did not respond to initial resuscitative efforts, resulting in the baby's death at 20 minutes of age. Antenatal ultrasound scans had shown anhydramnios and large fetal kidneys with numerous large fluid-filled cysts. The liver appeared normal and no other anomalies were seen. Both parents had a normal renal ultrasound scan. What is the MOST likely diagnosis?

☐ A Autosomal recessive polycystic kidney disease
☐ B Autosomal dominant polycystic kidney disease
☐ C Posterior urethral valves
☐ D Bilateral multicystic dysplastic kidneys
☐ E Meckel–Gruber syndrome

15.11 A term baby born after spontaneous vaginal delivery is noted to be pale. Full blood count shows: haemoglobin 5.4 g/dL, white cell count 15.1 × 10⁹/L, platelets 286 × 10⁹/L. The blood film is normal. The baby remains well and is transfused with packed red blood cells. A cranial ultrasound scan is normal. In order to establish the cause of the anaemia, the NEXT investigation should be which one of the following?

- [ ] A Abdominal ultrasound scan
- [ ] B Coagulation screen
- [ ] C Apt's test
- [ ] D Kleihauer's test
- [ ] E Bone marrow biopsy

15.12 A girl infant has profound hypotonia and required intubation and positive-pressure ventilation immediately after birth. She was born at term following a pregnancy complicated by polyhydramnios and reduced fetal movements. The chest X-ray shows small but clear lung fields. What is the MOST likely diagnosis?

- [ ] A Trisomy 21
- [ ] B Neonatal encephalopathy
- [ ] C Congenital myotonic dystrophy
- [ ] D Cervical spinal injury
- [ ] E Spinal muscular atrophy

15.13 A pre-term infant born at 25 weeks' gestation is now 36 weeks corrected gestational age and is screened for retinopathy of prematurity. Both eyes are found to have stage 2 retinopathy of prematurity. Which ONE of the following should you tell the parents about the baby?

- [ ] A No further screening or treatment is required and the visual prognosis is good
- [ ] B No further screening or treatment is required, but spectacles are likely to be required later
- [ ] C No further treatment is required at this stage, but further screening is necessary and the visual prognosis is likely to be good
- [ ] D Treatment is required with laser therapy or cryotherapy
- [ ] E There are retinal detachments, and visual prognosis is poor

Extended Matching Questions

15.14 Theme: Gastrointestinal diagnoses

A   Oesophageal atresia
B   H-type tracheo-oesophageal fistula
C   Meconium ileus
D   Malrotation
E   Hirschsprung's disease
F   Duodenal atresia
G   Anorectal atresia
H   Necrotising enterocolitis

For each of the following case scenarios, select the most likely diagnosis from the list above. Each option may be used once, more than once, or not at all.

☐   1.   Term baby with abdominal distension presenting on day 4. Rectal examination resulted in sudden release of watery faeces.

☐   2.   Pre-term baby, born at 29 weeks' gestation presented with early respiratory distress. Polyhydramnios was noted antenatally.

☐   3.   Term baby presenting with initial abdominal distension and intra-abdominal calcification on abdominal X-ray. A prolonged period of assisted ventilation was required subsequently.

15.15 Theme: Patterns of dysmorphology and congenital malformations

A   VACTERL association
B   CHARGE association
C   Trisomy 13
D   Trisomy 18
E   22q deletion
F   Noonan syndrome
G   Fetal alcohol syndrome
H   Goldenhar syndrome
I   Rubinstein–Taybi syndrome
J   Congenital rubella

For each of the following case scenarios, select the most likely diagnosis from the list above. Each option may be used once, more than once, or not at all.

☐   1. Term baby, birth weight 3.2 kg, facial dysmorphism with cleft lip and palate, heart murmur.

☐   2. Term baby, birth weight 3.9 kg, facial asymmetry with abnormal left pinna, hemivertebrae in cervical and thoracic spine, heart murmur.

☐   3. Baby born at 30 weeks, birth weight 700 g, microcephaly, complex congenital heart disease, congenital diaphragmatic hernia, facial dysmorphism, abnormal fingers.

MT–F Answers

15.1   Group B *Streptococcus* infection: A B

GBS is a Gram-positive coccus, which is a commensal in the gastrointestinal and genital tracts. It has several subtypes according to capsular polysaccharide antigens. Most neonatal infections are caused by subtypes I–III. Of babies born to colonised women, approximately 1% become infected. Approximately 10–30% of pregnant women are colonised with GBS. Although it can be passed on by sexual contact, it is not considered a sexually transmitted disease, as it is usually asymptomatic in adults. Benzyl-penicillin is the antibiotic of choice for neonatal GBS sepsis.

15.2   Anaemia in a newborn: A E

At birth, approximately 90% of haemoglobin is HbF, which consists of two α and two γ globin chains. Alpha-thalassaemia can therefore present in the neonatal period. The severity of this depends on the number of functional globin genes affected. The presence of no functioning globin genes is associated with severe hydrops and is incompatible with postnatal life; the presence of one functioning gene (HgH disease) causes haemolytic anaemia, and the presence of two or three causes no symptoms. Chronic feto-maternal transfusion may present with anaemia at birth, with diagnosis confirmed by a positive maternal Kleihauer–Betke test. Beta-thalassaemia and sickle cell disease do not present in neonates, with symptoms beginning at around 6 months of age. Glucose-6-phosphate dehydrogenase (G6PD) deficiency can present with neonatal jaundice. The haemolysis may be sufficient to cause anaemia within 1–2 weeks, but does not present with anaemia at birth.

15.3   Perinatal mortality: B D

Stillbirth is defined as in-utero death after 24 completed weeks of gestation. This definition varies in other countries, eg USA 20 weeks, Japan 18 weeks. The perinatal mortality rate is defined as stillbirths and deaths within 6 days of birth per 1000 live- and stillbirths. In England and Wales, it is approximately 8 per 1000. The neonatal mortality rate is the number of deaths of live-born infants younger than 28 days. This includes infants born at less than 24 weeks' gestation if live-born. Pre-term birth is the most common cause of neonatal death, accounting for more than twice as many as those associated with congenital anomalies.

15.4 Circulatory changes at birth: A D E

Functional closure of the ductus venosus occurs within hours of birth, with anatomical closure within a few weeks. Increased pulmonary blood flow, due to decreased pulmonary vascular resistance, which is partly facilitated by nitric oxide, leads to increased left atrial pressure, whereas right atrial pressure falls as a result of termination of blood flow from the placenta via the umbilical vein. This leads to functional closure of the foramen ovale. Decreased ductal sensitivity to prostaglandins and increased breakdown of PGE_2 occur towards the end of pregnancy.

15.5 Weight, fluids and skin: B

Normal weight loss after birth is due to extracellular fluid losses. There is a gradual decrease in extracellular fluid with increasing gestation (approximately 65% of weight at 26 weeks, 40% at 40 weeks). The surface area to weight ratio is high in newborn babies (more so in pre-term babies), so that the heat loss to heat production ratio is also high. Transepidermal water loss is increased for the same reason, and also because of the thin epidermis and stratum corneum. Sweating does not begin until approximately 36 weeks' gestation, so sodium is not lost along with water through the skin in very pre-term babies. Antenatal steroids have no effect on skin maturation.

15.6 Features of fetal alcohol syndrome: B C

Features of fetal alcohol syndrome include intrauterine growth restriction, facial dysmorphism, congenital heart disease (ventricular septal defect [VSD], atrial septal defect [ASD]), microcephaly with subsequent intellectual impairment, and postnatal failure to thrive. Maternal use of valproate (fetal valproate syndrome) is associated with neural tube defects, and maternal cocaine is associated with prune belly and other renal tract anomalies.

Best of Five Answers

15.7 D: DiGeorge syndrome

DiGeorge syndrome is a genetic defect caused by 22q11.2 deletion. The most common features are congenital heart disease (any, but most commonly aortic arch anomalies and conotruncal defects), cleft palate, absent thymus (low T-lymphocyte levels), and hypoparathyroidism leading to hypocalcaemia (and hence seizures). Renal anomalies are common, and there is facial dysmorphism (small mouth, and jaw and ear abnormalities).

15.8   B: Cytomegalovirus (CMV)

The clinical features described could be caused by either rubella, CMV or toxoplasmosis. However, routine vaccination has virtually eradicated congenital rubella in the UK, and congenital CMV is much more common than toxoplasmosis. Toxoplasmosis often causes hydrocephalus, and infection much more often occurs later in pregnancy. HIV does not cause an embryopathy, and affected babies are usually asymptomatic. Congenital syphilis may cause chorioretinitis, glaucoma, periostitis, hepato-splenomegaly and maculopapular rash.

15.9   A: Check urine for presence of ketones

Neonatal hypoglycaemia is defined as a blood glucose level less than or equal to 2.6 mmol/L. The key investigation is to check for ketones by dipstick-testing the urine. Ketotic hypoglycaemia may be the result of sepsis, adrenal insufficiency, panhypopituitarism, respiratory chain disorders, gluconeogenesis defects or defects of ketolysis. Absence of ketones suggests hyperinsulinism, fat oxidation defects or liver failure.

15.10   D: Bilateral multicystic dysplastic kidneys

The pathophysiology in this case is severe fetal renal dysfunction, from as early as the second trimester, leading to anuria and subsequent anhydramnios, resulting in severe pulmonary hypoplasia. All the listed diagnoses can have this effect. Autosomal recessive (infantile) polycystic kidney disease usually leads to large echo-bright kidneys on antenatal ultrasound scan, rather than macrocysts, and congenital hepatic fibrosis may be found. Autosomal dominant (adult) polycystic kidney disease usually presents later in life, but may rarely be a cause of microcystic changes within the fetal kidneys. Posterior urethral valves are associated with bladder and renal tract dilatation. Meckel–Gruber syndrome is another cause of fetal renal cysts, but other abnormalities, including encephalocoele, polydactyly, cardiac disease and liver disease are also found on antenatal ultrasound scan.

15.11   D: Kleihauer's test

The most likely diagnosis is feto-maternal bleed leading to anaemia. This can be acute or chronic. The Kleihauer (Kleihauer–Betke) test is performed on maternal blood and detects the presence of fetal red blood cells, thus confirming or refuting the diagnosis of a feto-maternal bleed. Apt's test is used if there is gastrointestinal bleeding, to distinguish between maternal and baby's blood as the cause.

15.12 C: Congenital myotonic dystrophy

All the options can cause neonatal hypotonia. Reduced fetal movements and polyhydramnios (as a result of reduced fetal swallowing) suggest a severe neuromuscular disorder. The small lung fields and ventilatory requirement suggest pulmonary hypoplasia, which may be secondary to severe neuromuscular disorders, which have an early in-utero onset (caused by reduced fetal breathing movements). This makes neonatal encephalopathy and cervical spine injury unlikely, because both of these nearly always occur secondary to an insult close to the time of birth. Although cases of spinal muscular atrophy with fetal onset have been described, they are extremely rare. Congenital myotonic dystrophy is therefore the best answer.

15.13 C: No further treatment is required at this stage, but further screening is necessary and the visual prognosis is likely to be good

The main risk factors for retinopathy of prematurity (ROP) are prematurity and hyperoxia. All pre-term infants born before 32 weeks' gestation and/or of 1500 g birth weight should be screened from 6 weeks of age. Staging determines treatment and prognosis, and reflects the degree of neovascularisation. ROP stages 1 and 2 usually regress, but continued screening is required until vascularisation is complete. Visual prognosis is good, but there is an increased risk of refractive errors and squint. Stage 3 ROP usually regresses, but requires close observation until vascularisation is complete, as treatment with laser or cryotherapy may be required. There is a high incidence of refractive errors and squint. ROP stages 4 and 5 involve sub-total and total retinal detachment, usually with poor visual prognosis.

EMQ Answers

15.14 Gastrointestinal diagnoses

1. E: Hirschsprung's disease

Hirschsprung's disease may present with delayed passage of meconium, bowel obstruction relieved by rectal examination, enterocolitis, or later constipation.

2. A: Oesophageal atresia

Oesophageal atresia (with or without tracheo-oesophageal fistula) presents with polyhydramnios, and this often results in pre-term birth. Early respiratory distress is common; alternatively, respiratory distress may present after a few hours, with vomiting or choking on feeds. Other congenital abnormalities are common. H-type tracheo-oesophageal fistula is much less common and presents later in the neonatal period with choking and signs of respiratory distress, or later recurrent respiratory tract infections. Duodenal atresia is often associated with other congenital anomalies and presents with bilious vomiting, with diagnosis confirmed by a 'double-bubble' appearance on abdominal X-ray.

3. C: Meconium ileus

Approximately 10–15% of cases of cystic fibrosis present in neonates with meconium ileus, and over 90% of babies with meconium ileus have cystic fibrosis. Abdominal distension occurs as a result of intestinal obstruction postnatally, or there may be antenatal perforation leading to intra-abdominal calcification. Malrotation occurs as a result of incomplete rotation of the fetal midgut, and presents postnatally with bilious vomiting or sudden collapse, with acute abdominal signs if associated with midgut volvulus.

15.15 Patterns of dysmorphology and congenital malformations

1. C: Trisomy 13

Features of trisomy 13 include holoprosencephaly, scalp defects, micro-ophthalmia, cleft lip and palate, polydactyly, renal abnormalities and congenital heart disease.

2. H: Goldenhar syndrome

Features of Goldenhar syndrome include facial asymmetry with abnormal ears, deafness, epibulbar dermoid cysts, vertebral abnormalities and congenital heart disease.

3. D: Trisomy 18

Features of trisomy 18 include symmetrical intrauterine growth restriction, facial dysmorphism, clinodactyly, nail hypoplasia, rocker-bottom feet, congenital heart disease, diaphragmatic hernia and renal abnormalities.

VACTERL association has the following features: **v**ertebral abnormalities, **a**nal atresia with or without fistula, **c**ardiac malformations, **t**racheo-oesophageal fistula, **r**enal abnormalities, and **l**imb abnormalities. CHARGE association typically has the following features: **c**olobomas, **h**eart malformations, **a**tresia of choanae, **r**etardation of growth and development, **g**enital hypoplasia in the male, and **e**ar abnormalities. The 22q deletion (DiGeorge or velocardiofacial syndrome) includes hypocalcaemia resulting from parathyroid gland hypoplasia, thymus hypoplasia (leading to increased susceptibility to infection as a result of T-lymphocyte deficiency), congenital heart disease and cleft palate. Noonan syndrome consists of facial dysmorphism (low-set ears, flat nasal bridge), a short webbed neck and congenital heart disease (pulmonary valve stenosis and cardiomyopathy most common). The features of fetal alcohol syndrome include prenatal and postnatal growth failure, mid-face hypoplasia, flat nasal bridge, thin upper lip, microcephaly and congenital heart disease. Rubinstein–Taybi syndrome consists of facial dysmorphism with hypertelorism and abnormal nose, with broad medially deviated thumbs and big toes and microcephaly. In congenital rubella, there is symmetrical intrauterine growth restriction, microphthalmia, cataracts, hepatosplenomegaly and congenital heart disease.

16. Nephrology

Multiple True–False Questions

16.1 Complications of nephrotic syndrome include:

- [ ] A hyperlipidaemia
- [ ] B malnutrition
- [ ] C primary pneumococcal peritonitis
- [ ] D prolonged bleeding
- [ ] E pulmonary embolism

16.2 The following suggest pre-renal, rather than intrinsic, renal failure:

- [ ] A urea of > 15 mmol/L
- [ ] B urinary sodium < 10 mmol/L
- [ ] C urine output less than 1 mL/kg/hour
- [ ] D hypotension
- [ ] E urinary osmolality of > 500 mosmol/L

16.3 The following is true of autosomal recessive polycystic kidney disease:

- [ ] A the gene for autosomal recessive polycystic kidney disease is found on chromosome 6
- [ ] B large renal cysts (> 2 mm) on antenatal renal ultrasound scanning are characteristic
- [ ] C it is always associated with some degree of hepatic fibrosis
- [ ] D it is associated with cerebral aneurysms
- [ ] E hypertension is an uncommon complication

16.4 The following is true of vesicoureteric reflux:

- [ ] A inheritance is autosomal dominant
- [ ] B it can be excluded on renal ultrasound
- [ ] C it does not cause nephropathy after 5 years of age
- [ ] D 70% of grade II reflux will resolve by 5 years of age
- [ ] E it can be demonstrated using a MAG-3 renogram

16.5 The following are indications for dialysis in acute renal failure:

☐ A creatinine of > 700 μmol/L
☐ B increasing hyperkalaemia not responsive to conservative treatment
☐ C hyperammonaemia
☐ D urine output less than 0.5 mL/kg/hour
☐ E metabolic acidosis not controllable with sodium bicarbonate

16.6 Nephrocalcinosis is a recognised complication of the following:

☐ A Williams syndrome
☐ B steroids
☐ C prematurity
☐ D furosemide
☐ E captopril

16.7 The following are recognised complications of chronic renal failure:

☐ A hypercalcaemia
☐ B iron-deficiency anaemia
☐ C secondary enuresis
☐ D delayed puberty
☐ E hypophosphataemia

16.8 Posterior urethral valves

☐ A are excluded by a normal renal ultrasound on day 1 of life
☐ B are rarely associated with chronic renal failure if corrected surgically immediately after birth
☐ C occur in both sexes
☐ D are associated with polyhydramnios
☐ E an intravenous urogram is the investigation of choice

Best of Five Questions

16.9   A 7-year-old boy presents with a 10-day history of purpura on his arms and legs. He has had 3 days of pain and swelling of his ankles and left knee but is ambulant. On examination he is apyrexial, his capillary refill is 1 second, pulse 100 beats per minute, blood pressure 105/80 mmHg. Urine dipstick shows blood ++ and protein +++. Bloods on admission revealed haemoglobin 13.2 g/dL, WCC 6.7 × 10⁹/L, platelets 273 × 10⁹/L, sodium 140 mmol/L, potassium 3.7 mmol/L, urea 3.0 mmol/L, creatinine 42 μmol/L and C-reactive protein < 2 mg/dL. Which of the following actions would be the BEST?

☐ A   Commence intravenous cefotaxime
☐ B   Commence oral prednisolone
☐ C   Advise bed rest
☐ D   Measure his protein/creatinine ratio on early-morning urine for a week
☐ E   Measure his serum creatinine monthly for 6 months

16.10 A 7-year-old presents with a 3-month history of severe intermittent left loin pain. There is no past medical history of urinary tract infection. On examination he is apyrexial, his blood pressure is 170/90 mmHg, pulse 90 beats per minute and he has a palpable renal mass on the left side. Urine dipstick is negative for blood and protein. Urine culture is negative. Renal ultrasound reveals significant left renal pelvis dilatation (antero–posterior diameter 20 mm) with normal renal parenchyma and a normal right kidney and renal tract. Which is the MOST useful investigation to perform next?

☐ A   Micturating cysto-urethrogram
☐ B   DMSA scan
☐ C   MAG-3 dynamic renogram
☐ D   Intravenous urogram
☐ E   Plain abdominal X-ray

16.11 A 5-year-old presents with a 2-day history of right-sided facial weakness. He has had headaches for 6 months. On examination he is drowsy. His blood pressure is 180/95 mmHg, pulse 100 beats per minute and he is apyrexial. He has a right-sided VIIth cranial nerve palsy and bilateral papilloedema. The rest of his cranial nerves are intact. Examination of his deep tendon reflexes reveals symmetrical hyper-reflexia in his lower limbs, with down-going plantars. He has a gallop rhythm, normal first and second heart sounds, an apex displaced to the mid-axillary line. There are no murmurs and no radiofemoral delay. Blood tests reveal the following: haemoglobin 8.3 g/dL; WCC 7.0 × 10⁹/L; platelets 293 × 10⁹/L; blood film, hypochromic normocytic anaemia only; C-reactive protein < 2 mg/dL; sodium 135 mmol/L; potassium 4.9 mmol/L; urea 11.5 mmol/L; creatinine 231 μmol/L; corrected calcium 1.79 mmol/L (2.2–2.7 mmol/L); phosphate 2.9 mmol/L (1.1–2 mmol/L); bilirubin 11 μmol/L (< 17 μmol/L); urine dipstick showed protein + , blood not detected; renal ultrasound showed two small kidneys with cortical thinning. The MOST likely underlying cause of these findings is which of the following?

- [ ] A Brain tumour
- [ ] B Coarctation of the aorta
- [ ] C Encephalitis
- [ ] D Haemolytic uraemic syndrome
- [ ] E Reflux nephropathy

16.12 A 14-year-old girl presents with a 2-day history of painless macroscopic haematuria. There is no family history of renal or hearing problems. Physical examination is unremarkable. Blood pressure: 110/70 mmHg; temperature: 37 °C; urine culture: no growth; renal ultrasound: normal; full blood count and clotting: normal; sodium 140 mmol/L; potassium 4 mmol/L; urea 5 mmol/L; creatinine 79 μmol/L; C3 and C4 levels normal. In clinic, 2 months later, urine dipstick shows blood + + and protein +. A hearing test is normal. What is the MOST likely diagnosis?

- [ ] A Alport syndrome
- [ ] B IgA nephropathy
- [ ] C Nephrolithiasis
- [ ] D Mesangiocapillary glomerulonephritis
- [ ] E Acute post-streptococcal glomerulonephritis

16.13 A 2-year-old boy presents with a history of chronic diarrhoea. His parents describe him as having a good appetite. On examination his weight is on the 0.4th centile and his height on the 25th centile. His blood pressure is 90/60 mmHg and pulse is 90 beats/min. Further examination is otherwise unremarkable. He is mildly dehydrated. Blood tests: pH 7.47; PCO_2 5.3 kPa; PO_2 10 kPa; bicarbonate 30 mmol/L (normal range 20–28); urinary sodium 3 mmol/L; urinary chloride 4 mmol/L; serum sodium 135 mmol/L; potassium 2.7 mmol/L; urea 3.2 mmol/L; creatinine 40 μmol/L; full blood count normal; liver function tests normal; plasma renin raised. What is the MOST likely underlying diagnosis?

- [ ] A Bartter syndrome
- [ ] B Conn syndrome
- [ ] C Cystic fibrosis
- [ ] D Münchausen by proxy by administration of diuretics
- [ ] E Renal artery stenosis

Extended Matching Questions

16.14 Theme: Tubular dysfunction

A   Bartter syndrome
B   Congenital toxoplasmosis
C   Cystinosis
D   Lowe syndrome
E   Nephrogenic diabetes insipidus
F   Insulin-dependent diabetes mellitus
G   Reflux nephropathy
H   Pseudohypoparathyroidism

For each of the following scenarios choose the most likely diagnosis from the list above. Each option may be used once, more than once, or not at all.

1. A 6-month-old girl presents with recurrent episodes of dehydration. There is a history of polyhydramnios during the pregnancy. She is on the 0.4th centile for weight, the 10th centile for length, and she is clinically 10% dehydrated. Blood pressure is 80/60 mmHg. Investigations show: pH 7.47; PCO_2 4.5kPa; bicarbonate 32 mmol/L; sodium 135 mmol/L; potassium 2.1 mmol/L; chloride 80 mmol/L; urea 5 mmol/L; creatinine 52 μmol/L; serum renin raised; urinary sodium 40 mmol/L; urinary potassium 50 mmol/L.

2. An 18-month-old boy presents with a 6-month history of polyuria and polydipsia. Examination reveals 2-cm hepatomegaly. He has swollen wrists and knees consistent with rickets. He is photophobic. Blood pressure is 100/80 mmHg. Blood tests show: pH 7.25; PCO_2 3.5 kPa; bicarbonate 18 mmol/L; sodium 130 mmol/L; potassium 2.7 mmol/L; urea 7.2 mmol/L; creatinine 120 μmol/L; glucose 4.3 mmol/L; calcium 2.2 mmol/L; phosphate 0.7 mmol/L; alkaline phosphatase 2030 mmol/L; thyroid-stimulating hormone (TSH) raised; thyroxine low; urine dipstick shows glycosuria and proteinuria ++; urine pH 6.2.

3. A 2-year-old boy presents with failure to thrive. There is no history of vomiting or diarrhoea. He had cataracts detected in the neonatal period. He has global developmental delay and hypotonia. Investigations show: sodium 135 mmol/L; potassium 3.2 mmol/L; urea 3 mmol/L; creatinine 60 μmol/L; glucose 4.2 mmol/L; phosphate 1.5 mmol/L; corrected calcium 2.35 mmol/L; serum pH 7.29; bicarbonate 15 mmol/L; chloride 108 mmol/L; urine pH 5.5; urine dipstick glucose +.

16.15 Theme: Hyponatraemia

A   Chronic renal failure
B   Congenital adrenal hyperplasia
C   Craniopharyngioma
D   Cystic fibrosis
E   Diabetic ketoacidosis
F   Excessive intravenous administration of salt-poor fluid
G   SIADH (syndrome of inappropriate secretion of antidiuretic hormone)
H   Urea cycle defect
I   Viral encephalitis

For each of the following scenarios choose the most likely cause of the child's condition from the list above. Each option may be used once, more than once, or not at all.

☐   1.   A 2-month-old boy presents with tachypnoea and poor feeding. He
         was born in good condition at 36 weeks' gestation by spontaneous
         vaginal delivery. On admission he weighed 5.0 kg. His respiratory
         rate was 80 breaths per minute and he had marked intercostal
         recession. He was clinically diagnosed as having bronchiolitis and
         started on maintenance fluids of 0.18% sodium chloride and
         4% dextrose at 31 mL/hour; 12 hours later he developed profound
         apnoeas requiring intubation and ventilation on intensive care. At
         this point he is well perfused and he is not oedematous.
         Investigations on admission to intensive care showed: serum
         sodium 115 mmol/L; serum potassium 4.2 mmol/L; serum urea
         2 mmol/L; serum creatinine 41 μmol/L; serum pH 7.19; serum PCO_2
         8 kPa; serum PO_2 8 kPa; serum bicarbonate 20 mmol/L; serum
         glucose 4 mmol/L; urine osmolality 400 mosmol; urine sodium 50
         mmol/L; urine potassium 40 mmol/L.

☐   2.   A 2-week-old white boy presents with a 3-day history of poor
         feeding. He was born at term weighing 4.0 kg. On admission he
         weighs 3.6 kg, has dry mucous membranes and cool peripheries;
         temperature 37.5 °C; respiratory rate 60 breaths/min and pulse
         170 beats/min. The rest of the examination is unremarkable. Initial
         investigations show: serum sodium 125 mmol/L; serum potassium
         6.9 mmol/L; serum urea 6 mmol/L; serum creatinine 60 μmol/L;
         serum bicarbonate 18 mmol/L; serum glucose 2.7 mmol/L; serum
         haemoglobin 17.0 g/dL; serum white cell count 18 × 10^9/L; serum
         platelets 370 × 10^9/L; serum C-reactive protein (CRP) 5 mg/dL;
         abdominal ultrasound normal; urine sodium 50 mmol/L; urine
         microscopy: no white or red cells seen.

☐ 3. A previously healthy 5-year-old girl was admitted to hospital following a 4-day history of profuse vomiting and diarrhoea. There is no past medical history of note. She is tracking along the 5th centile for height and the 50th centile for weight. Her weight 1 month prior to admission was 16 kg. On admission she is lethargic, her capillary refill time is 6 s, her temperature 38 °C and pulse 160 beats/min, and she weighs 15 kg (9th centile). Initial tests show: serum pH 7.31; serum PCO_2 3.5kPa; serum bicarbonate 18 mmol/L; serum sodium 137 mmol/L; serum potassium 3.2 mmol/L; serum urea 6 mmol/L; serum creatinine 80 µmol/L; serum alanine aminotransferase 50 U/L (normal 28–44); serum albumin 27 g/L (normal 30–45); serum glucose 3.8 mmol/L; urine sodium 4 mmol/L; urine potassium 102 mmol/L; urine osmolality 900 mosmol. She is given four 150-ml boluses of 0.18% sodium chloride 4% dextrose over the first 3 hours of resuscitation until she becomes well perfused. She is then started on maintenance fluids plus 10% correction over 24 hours (0.18% sodium chloride 4% dextrose with 20 mmol/L of potassium chloride at 120 ml/h). After 12 hours she becomes drowsy, so she is re-examined. At this point her capillary refill is 1 s, pulse 120 beats/min, blood pressure 130/70 mmHg, temperature 37 °C. She then has a prolonged generalised seizure. Investigations at the time of the seizure show: serum sodium 115 mmol/L; serum potassium 4.2 mmol/L; serum urea 4 mmol/L; serum glucose 5 mmol/L; serum lactate 7 mmol/L; serum pH 7.2; serum base excess –7 mmol/L; serum PCO_2 6 kPa; urine osmolality 100 mosmol; urine sodium 20 mmol/L.

MT–F Answers

16.1 Complications of nephrotic syndrome: A B C E

The mechanism of elevation of cholesterol and low-density lipoprotein (LDL) is unknown. Chronic proteinuria and steroid therapy can lead to muscle wasting, which can be masked by oedema. Loss of immunoglobulin in the urine and immunosuppression with steroids predisposes to infection, particularly pneumococcal. Loss of antithrombin III and protein C and protein S, dehydration with venous stasis, and increased blood viscosity cause an increased risk of thrombosis. Hypovolaemia due to shift of water from the intravascular to the interstitial space is common. Symptoms include abdominal pain and anorexia. If hypovolaemia is severe, acute tubular necrosis can ensue.

16.2 Pre-renal renal failure: B D E

In pre-renal failure the kidney tries to conserve water and sodium, hence urinary sodium is low (< 10 mmol/L). During intrinsic renal failure urine concentrating ability is impaired so urinary osmolality is usually less than 300 mosmol/L. Urea increases in renal failure of both types, haemo-concentration and during starvation so it is an unreliable measure of dehydration. Oliguria (< 2 mL/kg/h in a baby and < 1 mL/kg/h in an older child) could be due to either reason. A raised blood pressure, gallop rhythm, raised jugular venous pressure/pulse (JVP) and good peripheral perfusion suggest intravascular overload associated with intrinsic renal failure. Low blood pressure and poor capillary refill suggest a pre-renal cause.

16.3 Autosomal recessive polycystic kidney disease: A C

Large echo-bright kidneys, with or without cysts that are small (< 2 mm) are characteristic of autosomal recessive kidney disease. The severity of hepatic fibrosis varies from subclinical to overt liver disease, which is the dominant clinical feature. There are two gene loci for autosomal dominant polycystic kidney disease, the commonest of which is on chromosome 16, adjacent to the tuberous sclerosis gene. Autosomal dominant polycystic kidney disease is associated with cerebral aneurysms, subarachnoid haemorrhage, mitral valve prolapse and hepatic cysts. Hypertension is a major clinical feature and it can be very difficult to treat.

16.4 Vesicoureteric reflux: A D E

Vesicoureteric reflux (VUR) is 20–50 times more common in children with a family history of VUR. Grade I or II reflux cannot be excluded on ultrasound.

The investigation of choice is micturating cysto-urethrogram. Reflux nephropathy can occur at any age, especially if there is associated detrusor dysfunction, as in patients with spina bifida. Vesicoureteric reflux predisposes to urinary tract infection.

A MAG-3 renogram can be used to demonstrate VUR by scanning over the kidneys while the child voids after all the isotope has drained from the upper tracts into the bladder. For this test to be reliable the child must be old enough to have bladder control and to void on command.

16.5   Dialysis in acute renal failure: B C E

Creatinine itself is not toxic and takes days to rise, even when there is no renal function, so there is no absolute level at which acute dialysis is indicated. Haemodialysis can aid removal of low-molecular-weight toxins, such as ammonia or salicylate. Acute renal failure results in impaired excretion of hydrogen and potassium ions. Hyperkalaemia can result in ventricular tachycardia and ventricular fibrillation. Oliguria is not in itself an indication for dialysis, although volume overload and resultant hypertension unresponsive to diuretics are. Acidosis can be refractory to sodium bicarbonate. Side-effects of sodium bicarbonate are hypernatraemia and hypertension.

16.6   Nephrocalcinosis: A B C D

Nephrocalcinosis is usually part of a metabolic disorder. Nephrocalcinosis is common in distal renal tubular acidosis but rare in proximal renal tubular acidosis. Hypercalciuria can cause nephrocalcinosis. Hyperparathyroidism, vitamin D intoxication, Bartter syndrome, Williams syndrome, corticosteroids and furosemide cause hypercalciuria. At follow-up, 27% of infants born at less than 32 weeks and 62% of infants with chronic lung disease have nephrocalcinosis. Low birth weight, diuretic therapy, inadequate dietary phosphate and duration of oxygen therapy are risk factors.

16.7   Complications of chronic renal failure: B C D

The main causes of chronic renal failure in childhood are: renal dysplasia; reflux nephropathy; glomerulonephritis; genetically inherited diseases, such as Alport syndrome or nephronophthisis; and systemic diseases, such as systemic lupus erythematosus (SLE) and Henoch–Schönlein purpura (HSP). Phosphate retention leads to hypocalcaemia and secondary hyperparathyroidism and bone resorption. Reduced synthesis of 1,25 hydroxy-vitamin D_3 contributes to hypocalcaemia and leads to rickets. Anaemia is secondary to dietary iron deficiency, reduced red blood cell survival and erythropoietin deficiency. Polyuria is usual until glomerular filtration rate falls to end-stage renal failure levels (less than 10 mL/min/1.73m²).

16.8 Posterior urethral valves: All false

A normal ultrasound on day 1 of life does not exclude posterior urethral valves because hydronephrosis may not be apparent until urinary flow has been established. Posterior urethral valves are always associated with some degree of renal dysplasia and around 25% will end up with chronic renal failure or end-stage renal failure. Renal dysplasia is known to occur even if the valves are operated on in utero. The classic presentation is of oliguria and pulmonary hypoplasia. They are associated with maternal oligohydramnios. They are best diagnosed on micturating cysto-urethrogram. To visualise the valves, films must be taken without the urinary catheter in situ.

Best of Five Answers

16.9 D: Measure his protein/creatinine ratio on early-morning urine for a week

The scenario suggests Henoch–Schönlein purpura (HSP). Around 70% of children with HSP have some degree of renal involvement, usually just microscopic haematuria with or without mild proteinuria. Patients can develop nephritic syndrome, nephrotic syndrome, hypertension, or chronic renal failure, sometimes years after the original rash. Persistent nephrotic-range proteinuria (protein/creatinine ratio > 200mg/mmol) warrants referral to a nephrologist for consideration of a biopsy. Arthritis usually settles without treatment. Bed rest does not alter the course of the condition. Serum creatinine is an insensitive measure of renal involvement, although it is of concern if raised. Steroids are rarely used in HSP but have been used for severe abdominal pain and severe glomerulonephritis.

16.10 C: MAG-3 dynamic renogram

The patient is most likely to have pelvi–ureteric junction obstruction from the scenario presented. The investigation of choice is a MAG-3 (dynamic renogram) to determine if there is obstruction to urinary flow. The patient is hypertensive (95th centile for systolic BP is 106+ [age × 2]).

Hypertension of renal origin can occur by a number of mechanisms. It can occur when there is obstruction to urinary flow, as in this case. It can also occur because of reduced renal blood flow, either generally (as in renal artery stenosis) or locally (which occurs in renal scarring). Vesicoureteric flux with renal scarring from previous urinary tract infection is also a possibility, so DMSA and micturating cysto-urethrogram should be considered.

However, vesicoureteric reflux without urinary tract infection would not cause loin pain. Abdominal X-ray and intravenous urogram would be indicated if nephrolithiasis were thought to be the cause of his pain. Nephrolithiasis is rare in childhood and in the absence of microscopic haematuria.

16.11 E: Reflux nephropathy

VIIth nerve palsy is a recognised complication of hypertension in childhood. The child presents with symptoms consistent with hypertensive encephalopathy, such as drowsiness, papilloedema and hyper-reflexia. The anaemia, low calcium, proteinuria, and high urea, creatinine and phosphate are consistent with chronic renal impairment. Renal impairment can cause hypertension, or be as a result of hypertension. The cardiovascular signs are consistent with heart failure, which could be a result of hypertension. The absence of murmurs and radiofemoral delay makes coarctation less likely. Raised intracranial pressure could cause hypertension but would not explain the other findings. Recurrent urinary tract infections and vesicoureteric reflux are thought to cause renal scarring and reflux nephropathy.

Sometimes there is no history of urinary tract infection. This may be because the urinary tract infections have gone undiagnosed or because the renal abnormalities are congenital dysplastic renal malformations, which are indistinguishable from renal scars on DMSA and ultrasound scanning. Children with renal scars should have yearly blood pressure checks for life.

16.12 B: IgA nephropathy

IgA nephropathy can present as an incidental finding of persistent microscopic haematuria or with any of the renal syndromes. Prognosis is good although 10% will develop hypertension, proteinuria +/– renal failure with long-term follow-up. Alport syndrome, a hereditary nephritis, could present with a similar clinical picture. There are X-linked and autosomal recessive forms. Deafness around the age of 10 years, hypertension in mid-teenage years, and end-stage renal failure in the third decade is usual. Family members of children presenting with haematuria should be screened for microscopic haematuria and proteinuria. Nephronophthisis usually presents with polyuria/polydipsia, often with a normal urinalysis, and progresses to end-stage renal failure in the first decade. Acute post-streptococcal glomerulonephritis and mesangiocapillary glomerulonephritis could present in a similar way, but C3 is usually reduced. Typically, mesangiocapillary glomerulonephritis has persistently low C3, nephrotic-range proteinuria (protein/creatinine ratio > 200 mg/mmol), hypertension and progressive renal impairment.

16.13 C: Cystic fibrosis

The patient has a metabolic alkalosis with a very low serum potassium, the causes of which are: Bartter syndrome; pseudo-Bartter syndrome; aldosterone excess; renin excess; or diuretics. Pseudo-Bartter syndrome occurs when sodium and chloride are lost from extrarenal sites, leading to a secondary hyper-reninaemia. Causes include cystic fibrosis, congenital chloride diarrhoea, laxative abuse and cyclical vomiting. The serum biochemistry is the same as in Bartter syndrome (hypochloraemic, hypokalaemic alkalosis) but there are appropriately low levels of urinary chloride and sodium (< 10 mmol/L). Renin is released from the juxtaglomerular apparatus in response to reduced renal perfusion, leading to increased angiotensin II, which causes vasoconstriction and aldosterone release from the adrenals. Aldosterone causes extracellular fluid expansion by distal tubular sodium and water conservation. Sodium is reabsorbed in exchange for hydrogen ions and potassium. Hyper-reninaemic states, such as renal artery stenosis, can produce a similar biochemical picture to the scenario, but the patient is not hypertensive. Conn syndrome, primary hyperaldosteronism, also causes hypertension but there is renin suppression. Loop diuretics can produce a similar biochemical picture to the scenario, although there would be a high urinary sodium.

EMQ Answers

16.14 Tubular dysfunction

1. A: Bartter syndrome

The metabolic alkalosis and very low potassium suggests Bartter syndrome. This is due to an inborn defect in the N–K–2Cl transporter in the thick loop of Henle, leading to salt and water wasting. The resultant extracellular fluid (ECF) volume contraction leads to secondary hyperaldosteronism and avid sodium and water reabsorption in the distal convoluted tubule, and reciprocal potassium and hydrogen ion excretion into the urine. Crucial to the diagnosis is the finding of inappropriately high levels of urinary chloride and sodium.

2. C: Cystinosis

In this scenario there is glycosuria with normal serum glucose and metabolic acidosis with an inappropriately alkaline urine. This suggests there is a proximal tubular leak consistent with Fanconi syndrome. There are a number of causes of Fanconi syndrome, such as galactosaemia, mitochondrial disorders, tyrosinaemia, fructosaemia, Lowe syndrome, Wilson's disease, cystinosis and heavy metal poisoning. Cystinosis is an autosomal recessive defect in the transport of cystine out of lysosomes. It leads to a multi-system disorder. Early features include Fanconi syndrome, photophobia due to cysteine crystals in the cornea, and hypothyroidism. Renal failure occurs around 10 years of age if untreated. Diagnosis is confirmed by raised peripheral blood white cell cysteine levels.

3.   D: Lowe syndrome

The oculocerebrorenal syndrome of Lowe is an X-linked disorder characterised by congenital cataracts, hypotonia, intellectual impairment and renal Fanconi syndrome. Hypokalaemia is not marked. There is no specific treatment. Patients develop chronic renal failure in the second to fourth decades.

16.15 Theme: Hyponatraemia

1.   G: SIADH (syndrome of inappropriate secretion of antidiuretic hormone) secondary to bronchiolitis

The apnoeas are likely to be due to hyponatraemic seizures rather than impending respiratory failure. This patient has inappropriately concentrated urine in the face of very dilute plasma (239 mosmol). The plasma osmolality is is calculated by:

$$2 \times (Na + K) + (urea + glucose)$$

The normal range is 275–295 mmol/L. To diagnose SIADH there must be evidence of fluid overload as well as signs of volume depletion. As water distributes freely between the ECF and ICF oedema is not usually present. In SIADH an increase in ECF volume and reduction in plasma osmolality fails to suppress antidiuretic hormone (ADH) secretion and, if normal fluid intake is maintained, hyponatraemia develops. It is caused by surgery, or by pulmonary disorders, such as infections or positive-pressure ventilation, or by disorders of the central nervous system, such as meningitis or hypoxic–ischaemic encephalopathy. Treatment is to restrict water intake.

2.   B: Congenital adrenal hyperplasia

The inappropriately high urinary sodium in the face of hyponatraemia and hypovolaemia suggests an inability to reabsorb filtered sodium. Broadly, the causes of this are renal failure, aldosterone deficiency and administration of diuretics. The relatively normal serum creatinine makes renal failure unlikely, although creatinine takes hours to rise in acute renal failure. With the exception of spironolactone, most diuretics cause hypokalaemia. The combination of low sodium and glucose and high potassium suggests adrenal insufficiency, the causes of which are primary (such as congenital adrenal hyperplasia or Addison's disease) or secondary (such as pan-hypopituitarism or tumours affecting the pituitary, eg craniopharyngioma). The lack of cortisol and aldosterone in congenital adrenal hyperplasia leads to production of adrenocorticotrophic hormone (ACTH). ACTH acts on melanocyte-stimulating hormone receptors to cause pigmentation in skin folds. There are a number of forms of congenital adrenal hyperplasia, which can present at various ages in various ways. In classic congenital adrenal hyperplasia there is deficiency of one of the enzymes in the biosynthetic pathway of the adrenal cortex (21-hydroxylase deficiency). The continuing ACTH drive leads to the precursors being directed along the androgen biosynthetic pathway, causing virilisation. This presents with ambiguous genitalia in girls and a salt-losing crisis or precocious puberty in boys. Investigation involves karyotyping, serum 17-hydroxyprogesterone (the precursor of 21-hydroxylase), urinary steroid profile, and adrenal androgen levels. Acute treatment is with hydrocortisone and salt replacement.

3.   F: Excessive intravenous administration of salt-poor fluid

The initial history and investigations are consistent with gastroenteritis with 10% dehydration. Although serum sodium is normal there will be a total body sodium deficit, as diarrhoea and vomit contain large amounts of sodium (75 mmol/L). The slightly low initial potassium indicates that the distal tubule is reabsorbing sodium at the expense of potassium. The girl is resuscitated with the equivalent of half her circulating blood volume (40 ml/kg) of salt-poor fluid and she then receives further salt-poor maintenance fluid. This will correct her water deficit but not the salt deficit, resulting in dilutional hyponatraemia.

17. Neurology

Multiple True–False Questions

17.1   Cerebral palsy
- [ ]   A   is a term meaning developmental delay and learning difficulties
- [ ]   B   is caused by a perinatal insult
- [ ]   C   is a non-progressive condition
- [ ]   D   is associated with epilepsy
- [ ]   E   is usually associated with normal imaging of the brain

17.2   Brain tumours
- [ ]   A   are the most common malignancy of childhood
- [ ]   B   occur in increased frequency in Gorlin syndrome
- [ ]   C   most commonly occur infratentorially in infancy
- [ ]   D   are treated by radiotherapy in children under the age of 2 years
- [ ]   E   rarely metastasise outside the central nervous system (CNS)

17.3   Fragile X syndrome
- [ ]   A   is easier to recognise in adults than pre-puberty
- [ ]   B   is associated with microcephaly
- [ ]   C   commonly associates with attention deficit and hyperactivity
- [ ]   D   is screened for in autism
- [ ]   E   can be detected on routine chromosome testing

17.4   The following conditions are correctly paired with expected cerebrospinal fluid (CSF) findings:
- [ ]   A   acute disseminated encephalomyelitis and CSF lymphocytosis with increased protein
- [ ]   B   tuberculous meningitis and high glucose with raised protein
- [ ]   C   Guillain–Barré syndrome and normal cell count with reduced protein
- [ ]   D   fungal meningitis and lymphocytic CSF with low glucose
- [ ]   E   subarachnoid haemorrhage and xanthochromia after centrifugation

17.5 In acute disseminated encephalomyelitis

☐ A unilateral optic neuritis is seen more commonly than in multiple sclerosis
☐ B peri-ventricular changes are pathognomonic
☐ C a relapsing course is more common than in multiple sclerosis
☐ D the electroencephalogram (EEG) demonstrates excessive slow-wave activity
☐ E headache, fever and meningism are less common than in multiple sclerosis

17.6 Which of the following are true of neonatal and childhood stroke?

☐ A ischaemic stroke results in a motor deficit in around 75% of cases
☐ B it is about as common as brain tumours
☐ C it is commonly treated by thrombolysis
☐ D it has a risk of recurrence > 10%
☐ E the risk of occurrence is increased in children with sickle cell anaemia

Best of Five Questions

17.7 An 8-year-old boy is found at night making salivatory and gurgling noises. He is unable to speak, but seems conscious. His face is twitching on the left side. Which investigation is MOST likely to confirm the diagnosis?

☐ A Brain computed tomography (CT) with contrast
☐ B Brain magnetic resonance imaging (MRI)
☐ C EEG
☐ D Thrombophilia screen
☐ E Lumbar puncture

17.8   A newborn presents with a weak suck and weak cry. There is a fluctuating ptosis and hypotonia. The baby has attacks of apnoea. The mother has no medical history of note. The tests for anti-acetylcholine receptor antibodies are negative and there is a decremental response on repetitive nerve stimulation electromyography. What is the MOST likely diagnosis?

☐ A Transient neonatal myasthenia
☐ B Autoimmune myasthenia
☐ C Congenital myasthenia
☐ D Mœbius syndrome
☐ E Spinal muscular atrophy type 1

17.9   An overweight 14-year-old girl has complained of headache on awakening for several weeks. She has papilloedema. Her blood pressure is normal. Brain MRI is normal. Which investigation is MOST likely to confirm the diagnosis?

☐ A Sleep EEG
☐ B CT of brain with contrast
☐ C Magnetic resonance spectroscopy
☐ D Lumbar puncture with manometry
☐ E Visual-evoked responses and electroretinogram

17.10 The following signs are seen in a child with an ischaemic stroke: contralateral hemiparesis with face and arm more affected than the legs; horizontal gaze palsy and hemisensory deficits; language and cognitive deficits, including aphasia and apraxia; and homonymous hemianopia. Which artery is the MOST likely to be involved?

☐ A Common carotid
☐ B Middle cerebral
☐ C Anterior cerebral
☐ D Posterior cerebral
☐ E Posterior cerebellar

17.11 A 3-year-old boy presents with frequent falling. There is evidence of delay in motor milestones. He walked at 22 months. On examination, he has a shuffling gait and foot drop. He has difficulty climbing stairs. Serum enzymes are normal. Nerve conduction studies are normal. CSF exam is normal. The electromyogram (EMG) reveals denervation and paucity of movement. The MOST likely diagnosis is which of the following?

- [ ] A Type 2 spinal muscular atrophy
- [ ] B Parkinson's disease
- [ ] C Werdnig–Hoffman disease
- [ ] D Emery–Dreifuss muscular dystrophy
- [ ] E Kugelberg–Welander disease

17.12 An infant presents at age 4 months with hypotonia, weakness, and constipation. On examination, the pupillary responses are poorly reactive. Investigation reveals incremental response on rapid (20–50 Hz) repetitive nerve stimulation and abundant small motor unit potentials on electromyography. The Tensilon (edrophonium chloride) test is negative. What is the MOST likely diagnosis?

- [ ] A Spinal muscular atrophy
- [ ] B Congenital myotonic dystrophy
- [ ] C Infantile botulism
- [ ] D Congenital myopathy
- [ ] E Myasthenia gravis

17.13 A 10-year-old girl presents with headache. It is unilateral, pulsating, and rates 6/10 on the pain scale. The headache is worse on physical exercise and helped by sleep. Sometimes she experiences photopsias. There is often nausea. What is the MOST likely diagnosis?

- [ ] A Cluster headache
- [ ] B Tension headache
- [ ] C Hydrocephalus
- [ ] D Chronic paroxysmal hemicrania
- [ ] E Classic migraine

Extended Matching Questions

17.14 Theme: Antiepileptic medication

A   Gabapentin
B   Sodium valproate
C   Phenytoin
D   Clonazepam
E   Carbamazepine
F   Lamotrigine
G   Levetiracetam
H   Phenobarbital
I   Vigabatrin
J   Lorazepam

Select the most appropriate antiepileptic medication for the following children. Each option may be used once, more than once, or not at all.

☐   1. A 15-year-old boy seen in clinic who has had three witnessed generalised tonic–clonic seizures in the past 3 months.

☐   2. A 4-year-old girl seen in clinic who has had four focal seizures and has an area of cortical dysplasia on brain MRI.

☐   3. A 6-month-old with infantile spasms and a chaotic hypsarrhythmic electroencephalogram. Wood's light examination reveals several hypopigmented patches.

17.15 Theme: EEG patterns in epilepsy syndromes

A   Hypsarrhythmia
B   4–5-Hz poly-spike and wave discharges
C   Diffuse slow and spike wave discharges
D   Burst suppression pattern
E   Trace pointu alternans
F   Occipital spikes
G   Centrotemporal spikes
H   No abnormalities
I   Electrical status epilepticus in sleep
J   Unilateral temporal spikes

For the following epilepsy syndromes, choose the most likely EEG pattern from those listed above. Each option may be used once, more than once, or not at all.

☐   1. Juvenile absence epilepsy.
☐   2. Lennox–Gastaut syndrome.
☐   3. Landau–Kleffner syndrome.

MT–F Answers

17.1   Cerebral palsy: C D

Cerebral palsy is defined as a non-progressive disorder of movement and posture caused by a lesion to the developing brain. The insult can occur in the antenatal, perinatal or postnatal period. There is a higher incidence of seizure disorder. It is important to understand and to try to classify the different types of motor disorder. Although learning difficulties occur with increased frequency in children with cerebral palsy, they are not invariable, and are not part of the definition. The recent advances in brain imaging and better quality of MRI scans has allowed for the aetiology to be identified in many cases of cerebral palsy.

17.2   Brain tumours: B E

Leukaemia is the most common malignancy. Brain tumours are the second, occurring at a frequency of between 1 in 20 000 and 1 in 100 000 in different series. They rarely metastasise outside the CNS. There are a range of syndromes, including neurocutaneous conditions in which brain tumours occur at an increased frequency. It is therefore important in the assessment to include a thorough systemic inquiry and general examination. Supratentorial tumours predominate in infancy, especially astrocytomas. Infratentorial tumours are most common in children older than 4 years. Radiotherapy is rarely used in patients younger than 3 years, because of its problematic long-term effects on the developing brain. These include cognitive difficulties, seizures and hormonal problems.

17.3   Fragile X syndrome: A C D

Fragile X syndrome is caused by a morphological abnormality on the X chromosome, and is the most common inheritable form of learning difficulties. Facial features become more obvious after puberty, and there is often macrocephaly. The children have a long face, high-arched palate and prominent jaw. Macro-orchidism is another feature. Autistic features and hyperactivity are common. It is necessary specifically to request screening for fragile X in autism, as this is not performed on routine chromosome testing.

17.4   Cerebrospinal fluid findings: A D E

CSF is produced mainly by the choroid plexus. It should have a clear and colourless appearance. Normal values in a child are as follows: protein 5–40 mg/dL, glucose 40–80 mg/dL with a CSF to blood ratio of 0.6, cell count $< 5 \times 10^9$/mL. In tuberculous meningitis, the glucose concentration will be decreased, with a high protein and increased cell count. In

Guillain–Barré syndrome the protein can be normal or increased. Values peak between days 4 and 18. There are often oligoclonal bands that indicate local synthesis of immunoglobulin within the central nervous system. Oligoclonal bands can occur in multiple sclerosis, subacute sclerosing panencephalitis, and Lyme disease. Xanthochromia occurs, with cell counts above 500/mm^3. This is a red–orange coloration of the CSF that occurs after breakdown of red blood cells. Oxyhaemoglobin is released and can be detected 2–4 hours after a subarachnoid bleed. It remains for 7–10 days. Xanthochromic CSF also occurs in hyperbilirubinaemia, hyperproteinaemia, hypercarotenaemia, and with some drugs.

17.5   Acute disseminated encephalomyelitis: D

Acute disseminated encephalomyelitis (ADEM) is the term given to a process in which there is disseminated inflammation at several sites within the central nervous system, believed to occur at one point in time. Infections are often associated, especially those of the upper respiratory tract. Relapses can occur, and these are thought to represent part of the same acute immune process; the term 'multi-phasic acute disseminated encephalomyelitis' is used (MDEM). If, however, there appears to be a chronic immune process with relapses occurring in different sites at different times, a diagnosis of multiple sclerosis (MS) is made. There are many pathological and clinical similarities between ADEM and MS. In children, ADEM is diagnosed more frequently than MS. Some features help point towards ADEM as a diagnosis   unilateral optic neuritis occurs less frequently in ADEM than in MS, for example. MRI can be useful. In ADEM there is relative sparing of peri-ventricular white matter and follow-up scans can show partial or complete resolution, in contrast to MS, in which there may be new lesions. The EEG is frequently abnormal in both groups, with slow-wave abnormalities being a non-specific sign of the encephalopathic process. The correct diagnosis is important, as the risk of relapse and prognosis is very different in the two conditions. The best way to differentiate the conditions is the subject of current research.

17.6   Neonatal and childhood stroke: A B D E

Childhood stroke is as common as brain tumour, occurring in 2–13 in 100 000 children and in 40 in 100 000 neonates. Around half of children presenting with ischaemic arterial stroke will have sickle cell anaemia or congenital cardiac disease. Other predisposing conditions include immunodeficiency, homocystinuria and bacterial meningitis. In the neonate the pathology usually suggests an embolic aetiology. Venous sinus thrombosis is particularly common in the neonate, although it can occur at all ages. Haemorrhagic stroke can be caused by coagulopathies or structural lesions such as arteriovenous malformation. There has been an argument in favour of giving thrombolysis for ischaemic stroke within the first 3 hours, but very few children will present to a stroke centre for accurate assessment and management within this recommended time. Around 75% of children with ischaemic stroke have a residual motor deficit. They may also present with cognitive and behavioural difficulties. Modifiable risk factors need to be identified to prevent recurrence.

Best of Five Answers

17.7   C: Electroencephalogram (EEG)

This is the typical presentation of a child with rolandic epilepsy, also known as benign childhood epilepsy with centrotemporal spikes. It is also common to have brief daytime hemifacial twitching, with increased salivation. This is a common condition, accounting for about 15% of children with afebrile seizures. It can be recognised on clinical grounds and has a distinctive EEG.

17.8   C: Congenital myasthenia

The clues to the diagnosis of myasthenia are the fluctuation of weakness and the decremental response with repetitive nerve stimulation EMG. There are three main groups of myasthenic syndromes: the autoimmune form (often known as juvenile myasthenia), congenital myasthenia gravis (sometimes called genetic), and transient neonatal myasthenia. The last is caused by transplacental passage of antibody to the acetylcholine receptor in mothers with myasthenia gravis. Clearance of antibody can take 5 months after birth. Congenital myasthenic syndromes are a heterogeneous group and the defect can be presynaptic, synaptic or postsynaptic. It is important to remember these in the differential diagnosis of apnoea in the newborn. Spinal muscular atrophy type 1 involves degeneration of motor neurones. There is symmetrical weakness caused by denervation, with associated muscle atrophy. The neonate often will present with hypotonia, but the face is usually strong, with full movement. There is no loss of sensation. The EMG demonstrates a neuropathic reduced recruitment of voluntary muscle unit potentials. Molecular analysis is now used to make the diagnosis, and over 95% of cases have deletions in the survival motor neurone gene (*SMN*). Mœbius syndrome is characterised by bilateral facial weakness. There is often paralysis of the abducens nerve (VIth cranial nerve) associated with it.

17.9 D: Lumbar puncture with manometry

Benign intracranial hypertension is a headache syndrome showing increased cerebrospinal fluid pressure when measured during lumbar puncture, in the absence of mass lesion or dilated ventricles. There are usually normal findings on examination, except for papilloedema and occasional VIth nerve palsy. The condition requires close monitoring of visual acuity, as optic nerve damage can occur as a result of chronically increased pressure. Treatment can involve repeat lumbar punctures to remove cerebrospinal fluid, acetazolamide and analgesics.

17.10 B: Middle cerebral

Common carotid occlusion may be asymptomatic. Anterior cerebral artery occlusions present with contralateral hemiparesis involving the leg to a greater extent than the arm and face. There can be a contralateral grasp reflex and gait disorders. Urinary incontinence is a feature. Posterior cerebral artery occlusions involve contralateral homonymous hemianopia. There may be memory loss and dyslexia.

17.11 E: Kugelberg–Welander disease

The usual onset of Kugelberg–Welander disease is after 2 years; often, affected children have walked late. There is slow deterioration that results in scoliosis and wheelchair-dependence. Type 2 spinal muscular atrophy, Werdnig–Hoffman disease and Kugelberg–Welander disease are all forms of spinal muscular atrophy, each having degeneration in the anterior horn cell of the spinal cord, and in some cases the motor nuclei of the brainstem. Type 1 is the most severe form and can present with reduced fetal movements or neonatal hypotonia. Type 2 is of intermediate severity, but the children are usually unable to walk unaided. Muscle biopsy and molecular genetic studies for the *SMN* gene confirm the diagnosis. Parkinson's disease rarely presents in childhood.

17.12 C: Infantile botulism

The conditions listed can all present with peripheral hypotonia. Infant botulism most commonly presents at 2–6 months with the symptoms described. *Clostridium botulinum* is a Gram-positive spore-forming organism found in soil, agricultural products and honey. Respiratory failure can occur. The toxin is released and binds irreversibly to presynaptic cholinergic nerve terminals, disrupting the exocytosis of acetylcholine. Positive stool culture or isolation of toxin is difficult because of constipation. Management is supportive. Pupillary responses should not be affected in the other conditions. A positive Tensilon test would be expected with myasthenia syndromes. The EMG in congenital myotonic dystrophy may demonstrate myotonic potentials firing at high rates that wax and wane in frequency and amplitude.

17.13 E: Classic migraine

Headache disorders are common in childhood. This is a description of classic migraine with aura of flashing lights. Cluster headaches are more common in males, most often occurring in those in their late 20s, and rarely in children. Periodicity is the predominant feature of cluster headaches, with chronic episodes of headaches lasting for 2–3 months. There is usually no aura, and the pain is excruciating, often in the trigeminal distribution, and may be associated with lacrimation, sweating, ptosis and nasal congestion. Tension headaches are diffuse and bilateral, often described as pressing or a being like a tight band; auras are rare. Chronic paroxysmal hemicrania is similar to cluster headache, but the pain is usually in or around the orbit. The headaches last for a short time (5 minutes), but occur many times a day. Hydrocephalus can present as headache. This is usually worse in the morning. There may be associated gait abnormalities and cranial nerve signs, notably VIth nerve palsy and diplopia. There is often loss of fine motor co-ordination. Papilloedema is frequently present.

EMQ Answers

17.14 Antiepileptic medication

The identification of a seizure type and/or an epilepsy syndrome provides information on prognosis and guides the choice of drug treatment when this is deemed appropriate. It is always important to consider the safety profile of the treatment and available formulation. Monotherapy at the lowest dosage to achieve control is the ideal with any drug treatment.

1. B: Sodium valproate

For idiopathic generalised epilepsies, sodium valproate is usually the first-line choice of medication. The exception is in teenaged girls, because it is necessary to consider the risk of polycystic ovaries as well as teratogenicity. Lamotrigine would be preferred in this group.

2. E: Carbamazepine

Carbamazepine is first-line therapy for focal seizure disorders.

3. I: Vigabatrin

West syndrome is characterised by infantile spasms, hypsarrhythmia, and developmental delay. The first-line medications for these patients are prednisolone, adrenocorticotrophic hormone or vigabatrin. With an underlying diagnosis of tuberous sclerosis, vigabatrin is preferred.

17.15 EEG patterns in epilepsy syndromes

Of note in addition to the answers below, hypsarrhythmia is an important EEG finding with which you should be familiar. It forms part of a triad for West syndrome: infantile spasms, hypsarrhythmia and developmental delay.

1. B: 4–5-Hz poly-spike and wave discharges

Juvenile absence epilepsy begins in the early part of the second decade. Absences are less frequent but can be longer than in childhood absence epilepsy. Generalised tonic–clonic seizures often occur. The frequency of the spike wave discharges is often faster than the 3 Hz seen in childhood absence epilepsy.

2. C: Diffuse slow and spike wave discharges

Lennox–Gastaut syndrome is the best-known example of symptomatic generalised epilepsy. Multiple aetiologies have been identified, including tuberous sclerosis, cerebral dysgenesis and Batten's disease. Seizure types include generalised tonic–clonic, absences, drop attacks and myoclonic jerks. The characteristic EEG is general irregular 1.5–2.5-Hz sharp and slow-wave activity, with slow background. During sleep, bursts of sharp discharges around 10 Hz can occur.

3. I: Electrical status epilepticus in sleep

Landau–Kleffner syndrome is an acquired epileptic aphasia in which regression of language skills occurs. The EEG abnormalities can show multifocal spike or spike and wave in the temporoparietal region while awake, and frequent generalised spike wave discharges (ESES, electrical status epilepticus in sleep).

18. Ophthalmology

Multiple True–False Questions

18.1 The following present with a painful red eye:

- [ ] A juvenile rheumatoid arthritis
- [ ] B *Toxocara canis* infection
- [ ] C glaucoma
- [ ] D herpes simplex
- [ ] E toxoplasmosis

18.2 The features of acquired Horner syndrome in a 3-year-old child following cardiac surgery include:

- [ ] A mydriasis
- [ ] B ptosis
- [ ] C ipsilateral anhidrosis
- [ ] D normal pupillary reflexes
- [ ] E heterochromia iridis

18.3 The following are causes of congenital cataracts:

- [ ] A maternal diabetes
- [ ] B galactosaemia
- [ ] C varicella zoster
- [ ] D hypothyroidism
- [ ] E maternal steroids

18.4 Ptosis is a feature of

- [ ] A Mœbius syndrome
- [ ] B Kearns–Sayre syndrome
- [ ] C abducens palsy
- [ ] D collodion baby
- [ ] E Marcus–Gunn jaw winking syndrome

18.5 Risk factors for retinopathy of prematurity include:

- [ ] A birth weight less than 1000 g
- [ ] B female sex
- [ ] C blood transfusions
- [ ] D pre-term gestation
- [ ] E intracranial haemorrhage

18.6 Leukocoria is a recognised feature of

☐ A cataract
☐ B toxocariasis
☐ C retinoblastoma
☐ D Hurler syndrome
☐ E persistent hyperplastic primary vitreous

Best of Five Questions

18.7 What is the MOST likely visual field defect in a child diagnosed with craniopharyngioma?

☐ A Blindness in one eye
☐ B Homonymous hemianopia
☐ C Bitemporal hemianopia
☐ D Peripheral field defect
☐ E Central scotoma

18.8 A 2-day-old neonate develops a copious purulent discharge with associated lid swelling. What is the MOST likely causative organism?

☐ A *Chlamydia*
☐ B *Neisseria gonorrhoeae*
☐ C *Haemophilus influenzae*
☐ D *Staphylococcus aureus*
☐ E Herpes simplex

18.9 Examination of the pupillary light reflex in the left eye of a 7-year-old girl reveals an absent direct reflex and normal consensual reflex. These findings are MOST consistent with which one of the following?

☐ A Left oculomotor nerve palsy
☐ B Right oculomotor nerve palsy
☐ C Left Horner syndrome
☐ D Left optic nerve lesion
☐ E Right optic nerve lesion

18.10 What is the treatment of choice for *Toxocara canis* infection in a 3-year-old boy presenting with leukocoria. Fundoscopy reveals a large lesion close to the macula with marked inflammation.

- [ ] A   Cryotherapy
- [ ] B   Corticosteroids
- [ ] C   Laser therapy
- [ ] D   Observation
- [ ] E   Antihelminthic drugs

18.11 Viral conjunctivitis is MOST commonly caused by which of the following?

- [ ] A   Adenovirus
- [ ] B   Herpes simplex
- [ ] C   Paramyxovirus
- [ ] D   Corona virus
- [ ] E   Coxsackie virus

18.12 A 5-year-old child presents with acute-onset ophthalmoplegia of the right eye with associated proptosis and ptosis following a heavy head cold. The MOST likely diagnosis is which of the following?

- [ ] A   Orbital cellulitis
- [ ] B   Mastoiditis
- [ ] C   Cavernous sinus thrombosis
- [ ] D   Frontal sinusitis
- [ ] E   Cerebral abscess

18.13 The MOST appropriate test for assessing acuity in a 3-year-old child is which of the following?

- [ ] A   Sheridan–Gardiner test
- [ ] B   Standard Snellen chart
- [ ] C   Catford drum
- [ ] D   Preferential looking test
- [ ] E   Graded rolling ball test

Extended Matching Questions

18.14 Theme: Eye movements

A   Abduction of the right eye
B   Adduction of the right eye
C   Abduction of the right eye on upgaze
D   Adduction of the right eye on upgaze
E   Abduction of the right eye on downgaze
F   Adduction of the right eye on downgaze
G   Upgaze
H   Downgaze
I   All directions

For the three causes of disconjugate eye movements described below, select the position of the eye where diplopia is maximal from those listed above. Each option may be used once, more than once, or not at all.

☐ 1. Right-sided Brown syndrome.
☐ 2. Right-sided abducens nerve palsy.
☐ 3. Right-sided trochlear nerve palsy.

18.15 Theme: Drug adverse effects

A   Phenytoin
B   Amiodarone
C   Paracetamol
D   Ibuprofen
E   Ethambutol
F   Rifampicin
G   Vigabatrin
H   Corticosteroids
I   Insulin

Match the following adverse effects to the drugs listed above. Each option may be used once, more than once, or not at all.

☐ 1. Visual field defect.
☐ 2. Colour blindness.
☐ 3. Corneal deposits.

MT–F Answers

18.1 Painful red eye: A C D

The uveal tract consists of the iris, ciliary body and choroid. Anterior uveitis (anterior chamber and iris) and panuveitis are painful, whereas posterior uveitis (choroid) is painless, and therefore disease progression may be more marked prior to diagnosis in young children. Causes of posterior uveitis include infection by *Toxocara* and *Toxoplasma*.

18.2 Horner syndrome following cardiac surgery: B C D

Horner syndrome results from a lack of sympathetic innervation of the pupil. The pupil is constricted (miosis) with ipsilateral ptosis. Heterochromia is a feature of congenital Horner syndrome or early surgery involving the eye in the first year. Pupillary reflexes are normal.

18.3 Congenital cataracts: All true

Around 50% of congenital cataracts are idiopathic. The most common identifiable cause of congenital cataract is autosomal dominant inherited cataract, and therefore the parental history and examination need to be thorough. Other causes include maternal disease such as diabetes, and the maternal ingestion of exogenous steroids. Intrauterine infections (3%) and systemic disease (5%) account for only a small number of cases.

18.4 Ptosis: A B E

Mœbius syndrome results from a combination of facial nerve (VIIth) and abducens (VIth) nerve palsy and is often associated with an oculomotor (IIIrd) nerve palsy. An isolated VIth nerve palsy causes failure of abduction of the eye, but does not affect the lid. Kearns–Sayre syndrome is a mitochondrial disorder with progressive external ophthalmoplegia (reduction of gaze in all directions), ptosis, pigmentary retinopathy and heart block. A collodion baby is covered with a tense cellophane-like membrane resulting in ectropion as the tissues around the eyes are held in traction. The ptosis of Marcus–Gunn jaw winking syndrome resolves on mouth opening and lateral movement of the jaw. It results from aberrant innervation of the levator muscle of the eyelid from the trigeminal (Vth) nerve.

18.5 Retinopathy of prematurity: A C D E

Risk factors for retinopathy of prematurity include low birth weight, hyperoxia, respiratory distress syndrome, intracranial haemorrhage, pre-term gestation and blood transfusions. The incidence increases dramatically with birth weights of less than 1000 g. Adult haemoglobin dissociates oxygen more readily than fetal haemoglobin, so transfusions increase retinal oxygen dose. Gender is not a risk factor.

18.6   Leukocoria: A B C E

Leukocoria is defined as a white pupil and is indicative of an opacity at or behind the pupil (of the lens, vitreous or retina). The differential diagnosis includes cataract, retinoblastoma, toxocariasis, persistent hyperplastic primary vitreous, myelinated nerve fibres and retinopathy of prematurity. Hurler syndrome and the mucopolysaccharidoses – with the exception of Hunter syndrome – are associated with corneal clouding.

Best of Five Answers

18.7   C: Bitemporal hemianopia

Craniopharyngioma can be suprasellar, or supra- and intrasellar, and therefore as the tumour increases in size, pressure is applied to the optic chiasm. This is the site of decussation of the temporal field fibres and therefore vision in the temporal fields is lost bilaterally.

18.8   B: *Neisseria gonorrhoeae*

The very early onset makes *Neisseria gonorrhoeae* the most likely organism, usually presenting on day 2–4 of life. *Staphylococcus* and *Streptococcus* cause purulent neonatal conjunctivitis, but present later (day 4–7). *Chlamydia* produces a serous or purulent discharge (day 4–10). *Haemophilus* tends to cause a serous discharge (onset 5–10 days) as does herpes simplex, but the onset is much later (6 days to 2 weeks).

18.9   D: Left optic nerve lesion

The findings are consistent with damage to the optic nerve in the affected eye. In IIIrd nerve palsy the pupil is fixed dilated and does not react to direct or consensual light. In Horner syndrome the pupils are small due to the interrupted sympathetic supply to the pupillary dilator muscle, but are able to constrict to light.

18.10 B: Corticosteroids

The site of the lesion requires active management. Steroids are the preferred choice, either systemic or peri-ocular. Small peripheral lesions may be observed. The use of antihelminthic drugs is controversial as death of the larva can exacerbate the inflammation, and steroids would still be prescribed. Laser therapy has been advocated but it has the same increased risk of inflammation following death of the larva.

18.11 A: Adenovirus

Viral conjunctivitis is usually caused by adenovirus and is very contagious. First one eye is involved, and this then spreads to the other. Signs and symptoms include tearing, redness, and the sensation of having a foreign body in the eye. If the cornea becomes involved, then photophobia can develop.

18.12 C: Cavernous sinus thrombosis

The main differential diagnosis is between orbital cellulitis and cavernous sinus thrombosis. However, the latter is suggested by the acute onset of reduction in eye movements. The ophthalmoplegia is secondary to IIIrd, IVth and VIth nerve involvement, all of which pass through the cavernous sinus. Eye movements may be slightly reduced secondary to pain in orbital cellulitis. Treatment consists of intravenous antibiotics and/or drainage of sinuses if they are the source of infection. Frontal sinusitis presents with tenderness over the forehead and may be the source of the infection along with sphenoid and the ethmoid sinuses. Mastoiditis presents with swelling over the mastoid air cells behind the ear. A cerebral abscess is more likely to present with altered consciousness, vomiting and pyrexia.

18.13 A: Sheridan–Gardiner test

In the Sheridan–Gardiner test, the child has a key card with five letters. The examiner stands 6 m away and holds up letters of different size which the child has to match with those on the card. A standard Snellen chart can usually be used in children aged 7 years upwards. The other three tests are used for testing in pre-verbal children. The Catford drum (vertical stripes) relies on normal acuity to produce optokinetic nystagmus.

EMQ Answers

18.14   Eye movements

1.   D: Adduction of the right eye on upgaze

Brown syndrome results from a congenitally tight superior oblique muscle tendon complex. This means that the eye fails to elevate in adduction. Patients may develop a compensatory chin lift and may slightly turn their face away from the affected eye.

2. A: Abduction of the right eye

The abducens (VIth) nerve innervates the lateral rectus muscle, which abducts the eye.

3. E: Abduction of the right eye on downgaze

The trochlear (IVth) nerve innervates the superior oblique muscle, which acts to depress and intort (twist nasally) the eye. Patients usually present with head tilt to the opposite side. This is common congenitally or from trauma.

18.15 Drug Adverse Effexts

1. G: Vigabatrin

Vigabatrin can cause permanent visual field loss, and therefore an attempt should be made to assess baseline perimetry prior to – or soon after – starting treatment, and every 6 months thereafter.

2. E: Ethambutol

Ethambutol is used to treat tuberculosis. Retrobulbar neuritis is a dose-dependent side-effect that presents with colour vision defects, central and paracentral scotoma, and reduced acuity. Recovery can take weeks to months after ethambutol is stopped.

3. B: Amiodarone

Amiodarone deposits are seen in both lens and cornea, and are related both to dosage and duration of treatment. The deposits are reversible.

19. Paediatric Surgery

Multiple True–False Questions

19.1 Undescended testes:

- ☐ A should be fixed in the scrotum at 5 years of age
- ☐ B if impalpable, indicate that the testes have atrophied
- ☐ C if retractile, should always be operated on and fixed in the scrotum
- ☐ D if unilateral, will not affect the fertility rate
- ☐ E more common in premature neonates

19.2 Ingested foreign bodies

- ☐ A commonly get stuck at the level of the diaphragm
- ☐ B almost always need to be surgically removed
- ☐ C that become bezoars are easily removed from the stomach endoscopically
- ☐ D should always be viewed with a lateral as well as an anteroposterior chest X-ray
- ☐ E may be encouraged to pass into the stomach from the oesophagus by a trial of milk and bread

19.3 Testicular torsion

- ☐ A only occurs in postpubertal boys
- ☐ B can await its turn on the emergency operating list
- ☐ C can be intermittent
- ☐ D can be reliably diagnosed by Doppler ultrasound
- ☐ E of 12 hours' duration would suggest that the testis was salvageable

19.4 Meckel's diverticulum

- ☐ A is distinguishable from a gut duplication on radioisotope scanning
- ☐ B is implicated in small-bowel obstruction
- ☐ C is sited in the jejunum
- ☐ D causes bleeding by generating excessive acid in the stomach
- ☐ E presents with an umbilical discharge

19.5   Hypospadias

☐ A   describes an imperfect location of the urethral meatus in boys or girls
☐ B   is associated with inter-sex states
☐ C   is associated with abnormalities of the ureter or kidney
☐ D   is a heritable condition
☐ E   is associated with difficulties in coitus

19.6   Umbilical hernias in children younger than 5 years

☐ A   usually resolve spontaneously
☐ B   are not, typically, painful or tender
☐ C   are less likely to resolve spontaneously in Afro-Caribbean children than in white children
☐ D   become irreducible
☐ E   share clinical features with supra-umbilical hernias

19.7   Pectus excavatum

☐ A   is characterised by dyspnoea at rest
☐ B   is associated with chest pain
☐ C   is associated with congenital diaphragmatic hernia
☐ D   resolves spontaneously
☐ E   responds to physiotherapy

Best of Five Questions

19.8   A 1-year-old boy has a soft fluctuant swelling in the posterior triangle of the left side of the neck. This temporarily increased in size following an upper respiratory tract infection. What is the MOST likely diagnosis?

☐ A   Cervical lymphadenopathy
☐ B   Branchial cyst
☐ C   Thyroglossal cyst
☐ D   Cystic hygroma
☐ E   Parotitis (mumps)

19.9   A 5-year-old boy presents with a week's history of abdominal pain, diarrhoea and vomiting. On examination he is pyrexial, with a mass in the right iliac fossa. A diagnosis of appendix mass is made. The BEST treatment would be:

☐ A Immediate laparotomy
☐ B Resuscitation and laparoscopic appendectomy
☐ C Resuscitation followed by laparotomy
☐ D Conservative treatment with antibiotics
☐ E Ultrasound scan to confirm diagnosis, and conservative treatment with antibiotics

19.10 A 6-week-old baby with pyloric stenosis would be BEST ready for theatre when his electrolytes are (all mmol/L, except pH):

☐ A Bicarbonate 32   Potassium 3.4   pH 7.52
☐ B Chloride 97   Potassium 3.9   pH 7.49
☐ C Bicarbonate 18   Potassium 5.5   Chloride 110
☐ D Bicarbonate 22   Potassium 4.1   pH 7.40
☐ E Chloride 106   Bicarbonate 33   Sodium 138

19.11 An 18-month-old boy presents with vomiting, abdominal pain and rectal bleeding. He is dehydrated and there is an abdominal mass. A Meckel's scan is negative. What is the MOST likely diagnosis?

☐ A Enteric duplication
☐ B Intussusception
☐ C Meckel's diverticulum
☐ D Midgut volvulus
☐ E Appendicitis

19.12 An 8-year-old boy presents with abdominal pain and bile-stained vomit. A contrast study of the upper gastrointestinal tract reveals his duodenojejunal flexure is lying in the midline. No mass is palpable in the abdomen. Which is the MOST likely diagnosis?

☐ A Intussusception
☐ B Appendicitis
☐ C Colonic carcinoma
☐ D Midgut malrotation
☐ E Adhesion obstruction

19.13 A 6-year-old boy has a healthy prepuce, which is 60% adherent to the glanular surface. What is the BEST treatment?

- [ ] A   Divide the adhesions in outpatients
- [ ] B   Divide the adhesions under general anaesthesia
- [ ] C   Circumcise
- [ ] D   Allow for spontaneous resolution
- [ ] E   Use steroid creams

19.14 Inguinal hernias in premature boy infants are MOST likely to:

- [ ] A   Resolve spontaneously
- [ ] B   Result in testicular atrophy
- [ ] C   Recur after surgery
- [ ] D   Transform into hydrocoeles
- [ ] E   Be direct hernias

Extended Matching Questions

19.15 Theme: Radiological interventions

A   Ultrasound
B   Contrast enema
C   MRI
D   Air enema
E   Upper gastrointestinal contrast study
F   Oesophagogastroduodenoscopy
G   CT
H   Colonoscopy

For each of the following clinical scenarios, choose the most appropriate radiological investigation. Each option may be used once, more than once, or not at all.

☐ 1. A 4-week-old boy presents with a 3-day history of non-bilious vomiting. His blood gas is normal. Ultrasound shows a pyloric length of 16 mm and a muscle thickness of 4 mm, with the possibility of fluid passing into the duodenum. Which investigation would you perform next to make a diagnosis of pyloric stenosis?

☐ 2. A 15-month-old girl with 1 week's history of upper respiratory tract infection (URTI) presents with a 2-day history of irritability and non-bilious vomiting that became bilious. Ultrasound suggests a target lesion in the right upper quadrant. Which radiological intervention would you perform next?

☐ 3. A 10-month-old girl presents with a congenital midline cystic mass on the forehead. This is non-tender, with no change in size. Skull X-ray shows some scalloping of the frontal bone. Which radiological investigation would you perform next to make a diagnosis?

MT–F Answers

19.1   Undescended testes: D E

Undescended testis occurs when the testis cannot be brought down into the scrotum. Many infant boys have retractile testis, whereby the testis will come down into the scrotum but regularly retract upwards into the inguinal canal as a result of the cremesteric reflex. Retractile testes do not require an orchidopexy. Approximately 2–5% of newborn males have undescended testes; this reduces to 1.6% by 6 months of age. The incidence is considerably higher in premature babies. Orchidopexy should be performed when the infant is about 12 months of age. This allows enough time for any spontaneous descent, but is early enough to limit irreversible spermatogenesis. Twenty per cent of undescended testes are impalpable. This can be because of anorchia, atrophy or a high position (either within the inguinal canal or intra-abdominal). Fertility rates for a unilateral undescended testis are essentially the same as for the normal population, but fertility decreases to 50% for bilateral undescended testes.

19.2   Ingested foreign bodies: E

Ingestion of foreign bodies is very common in childhood. The vast majority of ingested foreign bodies will pass easily with conservative treatment. The most common sites of impaction are at the cricopharyngeus, aortic arch (4th thoracic vertebrae) and pylorus. The majority of foreign bodies are radio-opaque and visible on plain X-ray. If the foreign body is in the midline and is at or above the level of the carina, a lateral chest X-ray is required to ensure that the foreign body is not in the trachea. All batteries in the oesophagus, and those in the stomach for more than 24 hours, should be removed endoscopically. With all other foreign bodies in the oesophagus, provided the patient is swallowing their saliva and not drooling, a trial of oral fluid followed by bread and jam often encourages the foreign body to pass into the stomach. If this fails, then an oesophageal foreign body needs to be removed endoscopically. Gastric bezoars (trichobezoars) are usually very large and virtually impossible to remove endoscopically, and invariably require a laparotomy.

19.3   Testicular torsion: C

Testicular torsion can happen at any age during childhood. There are two ages at which the diagnosis of testicular torsion is more likely in a boy presenting with an acute scrotum: neonatal and peripubertal (peak age of 14 years). Neonatal torsion is an extravaginal torsion of the testis (testis and tunica vaginalis both twist en masse). This can happen both antenatally and postnatally up to 3 months of age. Torsion in older children is usually the result of an anatomical variant called the 'bell-clapper testis'. In this condition, the tunica vaginalis inserts high up the spermatic cord, allowing the testis to twist within the tunica. Torsion of the testis can be intermittent and these boys present with intermittent, severe testicular pain and, often, a transverse lie of the testes. These children need to undergo testicular fixation. An acute testicular torsion is a clinical diagnosis. Doppler ultrasound may help make the diagnosis by showing increased testicular blood flow. This is often seen in epididymo-orchitis, which is one of the common differential diagnoses of an acute scrotum. However, it is not reliable in excluding testicular torsion. Testicular torsion is one of the true paediatric surgical emergencies, and should always take priority on the emergency list. Whether a testis post-torsion is salvageable is dependent on the duration of ischaemia. A 6-hour history or less has a salvage rate of 85–97%. This drops considerably after 12 hours, with the potential concomitant risk of also developing auto-antibodies against the contralateral testis.

19.4   Meckel's diverticulum: B

Meckel's diverticulum is sited in the distal ileum, and is lined by ectopic gastric mucosa. The mucosa produces acid, which may ulcerate the adjacent diverticular and ileal mucosae, causing enteric bleeding or perforation. The ectopic gastric mucosa takes up and excretes technetium-99 pertechnetate, so can be detected by scintigraphy. However, false-positive results occur because this isotope also images duplication cysts and Barrett's oesophagus. The diverticulum may be connected to the umbilicus by a band of fibrous tissue, which may cause small-bowel obstruction. This band is the remnant of the omphalomesenteric duct. If the duct is patent, then a connection between the gut and the skin is formed, allowing umbilical leakage. However, in these circumstances the diverticulum is no longer blind-ended, and would therefore be defined as a fistula.

19.5   Hypospadias: A B D E

Hypospadias in boys involves a ventral urethral meatus, and is almost always associated with a hooded dorsal foreskin that is deficient ventrally. In addition, the ventral skin is often tight, leading to a bent erection. In girls, the term hypospadias refers to the recession of the urethral meatus proximally up the anterior wall of the vagina. Penile hypospadias is one of the major features of the ambiguity of the genitalia encountered in inter-sex states. Male hypospadias often runs in families, although Mendelian inheritance is only one of a variety of proposed aetiologies. Others include the ingestion of antiandrogenic medications (such as cimetidine) during pregnancy, and the ingestion of increasing amounts of oestrogens. Coitus may be difficult with a substantially bent erection. Hypospadias is not associated with upper tract pathology.

19.6 Umbilical hernias: A B D E

Both umbilical and supra-umbilical hernias present with a bulge in the umbilical region. The umbilical hernia tends to bulge outwards, through a circular defect in the abdominal wall. The supra-umbilical variety emerges from a linear defect and bulges downwards. Because umbilical herniation occurs through a circular scar, and scars almost always contract, the hole will close and umbilical hernias usually resolve spontaneously, given time. The process of closure may continue up to puberty, but if the child is teased about it, or at parental request, surgical closure can be performed. Surgical preferences vary widely, but there is some consensus for repairing the hernia when the child is 4–7 years old. The hernia can cause symptoms of discomfort, but rarely becomes irreducible.

19.7 Pectus excavatum: B C D

Pectus excavatum is strongly associated with connective tissues disorders, and with syndromes in which these disorders occur, such as Marfan syndrome. It is also seen often in survivors of repaired congenital diaphragmatic hernia. About 30–40% of patients with pectus complain of chest wall pain and tenderness. Pectus excavatum can resolve, although this is rare and it may be that many patients just simply become resigned to the presence of their deformity. For those in whom the condition does not resolve, surgery may be an option. There is little evidence that pectus deformities have any effect on cardiorespiratory function. The indications for surgery are therefore limited to the cosmetic and social problems associated with thoracic deformity. Minimally invasive pectus surgery is more likely to be considered by many adolescents who might have been discouraged by the invasiveness of the previously available open-repair technique.

Best of Five Answers

19.8　D: Cystic hygroma

Cystic hygromas are usually fluctuant and positioned in the posterior triangle. They often increase in size or become infected following an upper respiratory tract infection. All the listed diagnoses can give swellings in the neck. Cervical lymphadenopathy can be found in almost any position within the neck, but swellings are usually small, firm and mobile. Branchial cysts are usually firm, well-circumscribed masses. These are the remnants of the second branchial cleft and the most common site is the anterior border of sternocleidomastoid. Thyroglossal cysts are usually midline or slightly to one side, and would not be found in the posterior triangle. Mumps could be associated with an upper respiratory tract infection, but this would affect the parotid or submandibular glands, neither of which is found in the posterior triangle of the neck.

19.9　E: Ultrasound scan with conservative management

Children aged 5 years and younger are often diagnosed late with appendicitis, as a result of atypical presentations. Inflammation or perforation can result in walling of the appendix with omentum and surrounding bowel, resulting in a phlegmon or appendix mass. Performing a laparotomy in these children can be very difficult and hazardous. We now treat such children conservatively with triple antibiotics, initially using intravenous antibiotics and completing a total course of 2 weeks. Some form of imaging, usually an ultrasound scan, is performed on a clinically diagnosed appendix mass, because they can often contain pus (making them an abscess). An appendix abscess will not usually settle on conservative management, and requires some form of drainage. A child should never undergo surgery without adequate resuscitation.

19.10　D: Bicarbonate 22 mmol/L, potassium 4.1 mmol/L, pH 7.40

Hypertrophy of the pylorus results in an obstruction to the normal emptying of the stomach, and hence vomiting of gastric contents. This often occurs for several days before the diagnosis of pyloric stenosis is made, resulting in quite marked electrolyte losses and dehydration. There are large losses of hydrogen and chloride ions, with smaller losses of sodium and potassium. This results in a hypochloraemic, hypokalaemic metabolic alkalosis. Because of dehydration, the kidneys conserve sodium – and hence water – at the expense of hydrogen and potassium ions, further increasing the metabolic alkalosis. Also, the kidneys replace chloride with bicarbonate ions during tubular absorption of sodium, as a result of low chloride levels, which further potentiates the alkalosis. Babies with pyloric stenosis require resuscitation with an initial fluid bolus, followed by 150 mL/kg of 0.45% sodium chloride / 5% dextrose with 10 mmol potassium chloride to reverse the above process. The electrolytes, particularly the bicarbonate, should be completely normal before surgery is undertaken. High bicarbonate results in reduced hydrogen ions in the CSF, depression of the respiratory drive, and an increased risk of apnoeas post-operatively.

19.11 B: Intussusception

In this age group, intussusception is the leading diagnosis. A duplication cyst could give all these features, although it may contain sufficient gastric epithelium to produce a positive Meckel's scan. However, it would be a comparatively rare diagnosis. A Meckel's diverticulum is still possible (scintigraphy has poor sensitivity), and it could have bled, but there are also features of small-bowel obstruction. Although Meckel's diverticulum can be the cause of small-bowel obstruction, it is less likely to be bleeding and obstructing at the same time. Midgut volvulus is plausible and is important to consider in these circumstances. However, in this age group, it is less likely than intussusception. Acute appendicitis can certainly cause bowel obstruction and a palpable mass, but rarely presents with rectal bleeding.

19.12 D: Midgut malrotation

This boy has small-bowel obstruction. The abnormal siting of his duodenojejunal flexure (which should overlie or lie to the left of his left vertebral pedicles) indicates that, by definition, he has malrotation. This can lead to bowel obstruction, either by the predisposition to midgut volvulus, or as a result of the abnormal peritoneal bands that are inherent to malrotation and can obstruct the bowel, whether or not there is an associated volvulus. The lack of an abdominal mass makes the first three diagnoses less likely, although it does not exclude them. Acute appendicitis would be the most likely diagnosis if not for the results of the contrast study. It is certainly possible that a child with uncomplicated malrotation could get appendicitis. Intussusception is unlikely in an 8-year-old, and carcinoma (although it has been recorded) is very rare. Adhesion obstruction is a common cause of bowel obstruction, although absence of a past history of abdominal surgery reduces the likelihood in this child.

19.13 D: Allow for spontaneous resolution

Preputial adhesions resolve. All of the solutions described were still in use in the UK as recently as 2003. It is well recognised that, if preputial adhesions are separated by either physical or chemical means, the vast majority subsequently re-form. Smegma can accumulate under the adherent prepuce, forming a 'preputial pearl'. Once the adhesion resolves, this mass of secretions is extruded. Therefore preputial adhesions should be allowed to separate spontaneously.

19.14　C: Recur after surgery

Inguinal hernias in premature boy neonates have a substantial chance of recurring (in about 5–10% of cases). Inguinal hernias in children are nearly always indirect, the gut passing through the peritoneal channel made by the processus vaginalis. The direct form of hernia (a bulge through the posterior wall of the inguinal canal) is very rare in the absence of an underlying connective tissue disorder. Spontaneous resolution has been recorded, and would be expected to involve a transient transformation into a hydrocoele. The endpoint of the natural history would see the processus closing completely, leaving evidence of neither a hernia nor a hydrocoele. However, although both these situations are encountered anecdotally, they are relatively rare. If an inguinal hernia becomes incarcerated, it may damage adjacent tissues. The effects of local pressure cause damage of this kind. Pressure on the testicular vessels can cause ischaemia and atrophy of the testis. However, another cause of testicular vessel damage is the herniotomy operation needed to repair the hernia, which may prove to be a very difficult procedure. It may be impossible to identify which mechanism was responsible if testicular atrophy follows hernia incarceration.

EMQ Answers

19.15 Radiological interventions

1.   E: Upper gastrointestinal contrast study

Hypertrophic pyloric stenosis can usually be diagnosed clinically or by ultrasound (normal features are muscle thickness > 4 mm, pyloric canal length > 18 mm, and non-passage of fluid from the stomach into the duodenum). Upper gastrointestinal contrast is the gold-standard test for diagnosing pyloric stenosis when these less invasive investigations are equivocal.

2.   D: Air enema

This is highly suggestive of intussusception. An air enema will both confirm the diagnosis and be therapeutic in approximately 85% of cases.

3.   C: MRI

This is most likely to be a dermoid cyst. In this position there is a significant risk that it could be dumb-bell in shape with an intracranial extension. MRI is the most sensitive imaging technique with which to demonstrate this pre-operatively.

20. Respiratory Medicine

Multiple True–False Questions

20.1 The following are treatments for obstructive sleep apnoea in children:

- [ ] A leukotriene receptor antagonist
- [ ] B long-acting β₂-agonist
- [ ] C nasal continuous positive airway pressure (CPAP)
- [ ] D adenotonsillectomy
- [ ] E slow-release oral theophylline

20.2 Clinical manifestations of accidental hydrocarbon ingestion include:

- [ ] A fever
- [ ] B cyanosis
- [ ] C coughing and vomiting
- [ ] D dyspnoea
- [ ] E convulsions

20.3 Micro-organisms commonly infecting the airways in cystic fibrosis are:

- [ ] A *Stenotrophomonas maltophilia*
- [ ] B *Streptococcus pneumoniae*
- [ ] C *Mycobacterium tuberculosis*
- [ ] D atypical mycobacteria
- [ ] E *Burkholderia cepacia* complex

20.4 The following lung function changes are likely to be found in a child with neuromuscular disease:

- [ ] A decreased transfer factor for carbon monoxide
- [ ] B increased peak expiratory flow rate
- [ ] C decreased forced expiratory volume in the first second (FEV_1)
- [ ] D increased vital capacity (VC)
- [ ] E decreased FEV_1 to FVC ratio

20.5   The oxyhaemoglobin dissociation curve is shifted to the right in the following situations:

- [ ] A   increase in temperature
- [ ] B   hypocarbia
- [ ] C   alkalosis
- [ ] D   increase in D-2,3-diphosphoglycerate
- [ ] E   carbon monoxide poisoning

20.6   Lung compliance in infants

- [ ] A   is defined as the volume change per unit of pressure
- [ ] B   increases with age
- [ ] C   is increased in respiratory distress syndrome
- [ ] D   is independent of lung volume
- [ ] E   is dependent on type II pneumocytes

Best of Five Questions

20.7   A neonate born at 32 weeks' gestation develops respiratory distress in the first few hours of life. Which is the LEAST likely diagnosis?

- [ ] A   Spontaneous pneumothorax
- [ ] B   Patent ductus arteriosus
- [ ] C   Hyaline membrane disease
- [ ] D   Group B streptococcal sepsis
- [ ] E   Cyanotic heart disease

20.8   Parents come to you for antenatal counselling: the mother is a carrier of a cystic fibrosis mutation and the father, who is of white ethnicity, has never been tested and has no family history. Which ONE of the following is the chance that their child could have cystic fibrosis?

- [ ] A   1 in 4
- [ ] B   1 in 100
- [ ] C   1 in 160
- [ ] D   1 in 200
- [ ] E   1 in 2500

20.9 A 2-year-old boy has a history of lethargy and falling asleep during the day. His mother reports that he snores loudly. Which is the MOST useful investigation?

☐ A Arterial blood-gas analysis
☐ B Electrocardiogram (ECG)
☐ C Microlaryngobronchoscopy (MLB)
☐ D Overnight oxygen saturation recording
☐ E Lateral upper airways X-ray

20.10 A 14-month-old girl with a history of eczema develops generalised urticaria, wheeze and severe dyspnoea shortly after eating some peanut butter for the first time. What is the MOST appropriate initial treatment if she presents to her GP practice?

☐ A Adrenaline intramuscularly
☐ B Adrenaline intravenously
☐ C Hydrocortisone intravenously
☐ D Chlorpheniramine intravenously
☐ E Chlorpheniramine orally

20.11 A 10-year-old boy who was previously well presents with a 2-week history of malaise and headache, with pleuritic chest pain, cough and fever over the past 3 days. Five days of treatment with oral penicillin has brought about no improvement. On examination there is a small area of dullness at the right lung base and bronchial breathing in the right mid-zone. The MOST likely diagnosis is which of the following?

☐ A Lymphoma
☐ B *Mycoplasma pneumoniae* pneumonia
☐ C Pneumococcal pneumonia
☐ D *Pneumocystis carinii* pneumonia
☐ E Staphylococcal pneumonia

20.12 A 3-month-old baby has a history of wheeze and coughing, usually after feeds, since birth. Her weight is normal and on examination she has a Harrison sulcus and a hyper-expanded chest. Which of the following investigations would be the MOST useful?

☐ A Flexible bronchoscopy
☐ B Computed tomography (CT) scan of the chest
☐ C Ciliary brushing for motility
☐ D Sweat electrolytes
☐ E pH study

20.13 An 18-month-old girl presents with a 6-month history of weight loss and cough. Examination reveals a clear chest and red, tender lesions on her shins. Chest X-ray shows right upper lobe consolidation. Which is the MOST useful diagnostic test?

- [ ] A Erythrocyte sedimentation rate (ESR)
- [ ] B Bronchoalveolar lavage
- [ ] C Sputum culture
- [ ] D Gastric aspirate cultures
- [ ] E Skin biopsy

Extended Matching Questions

20.14 Theme: Management of pleural infection

A Repeated thoracocentesis
B Lateral chest X-ray
C Insertion of a large-bore chest drain
D Intrapleural fibrinolytics
E Ultrasound scan of the chest
F Insertion of a small pigtail chest drain
G CT scan of the chest
H Posterolateral thoracotomy with decortication

For each of the following scenarios, select the most appropriate management from the list above. Each option may be used once, more than once, or not at all.

- [ ] 1. A 5-year-old boy who is admitted to hospital in a tertiary centre for intravenous antibiotics because of a bacterial pneumonia fails to improve after 48 hours of therapy and needs oxygen supplementation. On physical examination, you find decreased chest expansion, dullness to percussion, and reduced breath sounds on the right side and you suspect a pleural effusion. Which of the above is the most appropriate imaging investigation?
- [ ] 2. The investigations you have performed confirm the presence of a large pleural effusion. Which next therapeutic step is most appropriate?
- [ ] 3. The pleural fluid that has been collected is yellow-greenish and thick. Which next therapeutic step is adequate?

20.15 Theme: Investigation of children with respiratory disease

A Sputum bacteriology
B Nasal brushing
C Bronchoalveolar lavage
D Lateral neck X-ray
E Barium swallow
F Rigid bronchoscopy
G Serum total and *Aspergillus*-specific IgE
H Flow–volume loop
I Serum viral studies

For each of the following case scenarios, select the most useful investigation from the list above. Each option may be used once, more than once, or not at all.

☐ 1. A 10-year-old boy with cystic fibrosis has a 1-month history of increasing wheeze and breathlessness. Chest X-ray shows a wedge-shaped shadow in the right mid-zone. Forced expiratory volume in the first second (FEV_1) is 65% of predicted (previously 98%).

☐ 2. A 2-year-old boy presents with a 2-day history of a persistent dry cough. On examination he has right-sided monophonic wheeze. Chest X-ray shows a hyper-lucent right lung, and the liver displaced downwards.

☐ 3. A 5-month-old girl with HIV infection presents with a 1-week history of fever, cough and dyspnoea. On examination there are crackles throughout her chest. Oxygen saturation is 85%. Chest X-ray shows bilateral diffuse shadowing. Nasopharyngeal aspirates for bacteria, viruses and fungi are normal.

MT–F Answers

20.1   Treatment for obstructive sleep apnoea: A C D

Obstructive sleep apnoea is a common problem in children and is characterised by upper airway obstruction that disrupts sleep. It can lead to impaired daytime performance and morning headaches, in addition to more serious complications such as heart failure, developmental delay and poor growth. Because adenotonsillar hyperplasia is the most common condition associated with paediatric obstructive sleep apnoea, adenotonsillectomy provides definitive relief of obstruction in the majority of patients. Medical management with non-invasive continuous positive airway pressure (CPAP) is an option in children in whom adenotonsillectomy fails. Pharmacological management has only a limited role: snoring associated with nasal obstruction can be treated with nasal decongestants and topical steroids, but this is rarely sufficient to reverse significant obstructive sleep apnoea. Recently, leukotriene antagonists, either alone or as part of combined anti-inflammatory strategies, have been shown to be effective in the management of children with sleep-disordered breathing that is too mild to justify referral for adenotonsillectomy.

20.2   Clinical manifestations of hydrocarbon ingestion: All true

Hydrocarbons, such as furniture polish, kerosene, charcoal lighter fluid and petrol are occasionally accidentally ingested by young children. Coughing and vomiting follow ingestion almost immediately. Hydrocarbons are probably aspirated during swallowing or vomiting, and can cause chemical pneumonitis, with fever occurring within hours, and dyspnoea, hypoxaemia and cyanosis. Systemic symptoms of hydrocarbon ingestion include somnolence, convulsions and coma. Supportive measures, including oxygen, physiotherapy and, if necessary, ventilatory assistance, are important components of therapy. Antibiotics and corticosteroids are not recommended.

20.3   Micro-organisms in cystic fibrosis lung disease: A D E

Cystic fibrosis is a major cause of severe chronic lung disease in children. Chronic infection of the endobronchial spaces of the airways in cystic fibrosis is mainly due to a failure to clear inhaled bacteria promptly, leading to persistent colonisation and sustained inflammation. Organisms typically infecting the airways in cystic fibrosis include *Stenotrophomonas maltophilia*, atypical mycobacteria, *Burkholderia cepacia* complex, *Staphylococcus aureus*, *Haemophilus influenzae* and *Pseudomonas aeruginosa*. *S. pneumoniae* is not common, neither is *Mycobacterium tuberculosis*.

20.4   Lung function in neuromuscular disease: C

As a result of inspiratory muscle weakness, scoliosis, and chest-wall stiffness, decreases in vital capacity (VC) and total lung capacity are typically observed in patients with neuromuscular disease. Peak expiratory flow rate (PEFR) and forced expiratory volume in the first second (FEV_1) are usually also diminished as a consequence of both decreased expiratory muscle strength and low lung volumes. However, as is the case in most restrictive lung diseases, the FEV_1 to FVC ratio is normal in patients with neuromuscular disease. Gas exchange, and therefore transfer factor for carbon monoxide, are also normal in these patients.

20.5   Oxyhaemoglobin dissociation curve: A D

The affinity of haemoglobin for oxygen increases as the partial pressure of oxygen in arterial blood increases. This is shown as a sigmoid-shaped plot of haemoglobin saturation against partial pressure of oxygen (the oxyhaemoglobin dissociation curve). The flat upper portion allows arterial oxygen content to stay high despite variations in PO_2. The steep middle portion of the curve describes how peripheral tissues (with a lower partial pressure of oxygen) can withdraw large amounts of oxygen from haemoglobin for only a small decrease in capillary PO_2. A variety of conditions can alter the binding affinity of haemoglobin for oxygen, thus shifting the curve left or right. Increases in temperature, carbon dioxide partial pressure, hydrogen ion concentration, and D-2,3-diphospho-glycerate all shift the curve to the right, facilitating removal of oxygen from the blood by peripheral tissues, as the affinity of haemoglobin for oxygen decreases. Opposite changes and the presence of fetal haemoglobin result in a left-shifted curve.

20.6   Lung compliance: A B E

Lung compliance is defined as the change in lung volume per unit of pressure. It is also represented by the slope of the pressure–volume curve. This has a sigmoid shape, so compliance also depends on the initial lung volume, from which the change in volume was measured (eg at large lung volumes at which the lung is near its elastic limit, the pressure–volume curve is less steep and hence compliance is reduced). Pulmonary surfactant produced by type II pneumocytes in newborns reduces surface tension and increases compliance. In respiratory distress syndrome, there is a deficiency of surfactant (most commonly as a result of prematurity) and compliance is reduced.

Best of Five Answers

20.7   B: Patent ductus arteriosus

Hyaline membrane disease (surfactant deficiency), group B streptococcal sepsis, cyanotic heart disease (eg total anomalous pulmonary venous return), aspiration syndromes, spontaneous pneumothorax, pleural effusions, or congenital anomalies such as cystic adenomatoid malformation or diaphragmatic hernia can all present with severe respiratory distress in the first hours of life. Although a patent ductus arteriosus can result in respiratory distress following left heart failure with pulmonary oedema, this usually does not occur within the first days of life.

20.8   B: 1 in 100

This question illustrates the commonly examined topic of inheritance. You will be expected to know the carrier frequency (1/25) and the prevalence in the general population of cystic fibrosis (1/2500) and other common conditions. We know the mother is a carrier and the father has a 1/25 chance of being a carrier, so the calculation $1 \times 1/25 \times 1/4 = 1/100$ gives the odds per pregnancy of producing a child with cystic fibrosis. The abnormal gene codes for cystic fibrosis transmembrane conductance regulator (CFTR), the main role of which is as a cyclic AMP-dependent chloride ion channel. Defects in CFTR in the lung result in reduced chloride secretion and hyperabsorption of sodium ions (and water), leading to viscid secretions. Remember that CFTR works in reverse in the skin, leading to failure to reabsorb sweat electrolytes – the basis of the sweat test.

20.9   D: Overnight oxygen saturation recording

This child has a history suggestive of sleep apnoea. The presentation can be subtle, and families will often not report pauses in a child's breathing while asleep unless specifically questioned. Other features that are suggestive are early morning headaches (due to high arterial CO_2 partial pressure [PCO_2]) and an 'adenoidal' voice. Sleep apnoea is most often caused by adenotonsillar hypertrophy, but neuromuscular conditions must also be considered. Arterial blood-gas analysis may show high PCO_2 and upper airway X-ray or MLB may reveal large adenoids, but most information will be obtained from overnight oxygen saturation monitoring. This will detect periods of desaturation and apnoea, and, linked to analysis of chest and abdominal movements, can help distinguish between obstructive causes (tonsils) and central causes (eg brainstem tumour).

20.10 A: Adrenaline intramuscularly

The history clearly describes an episode of anaphylaxis. Adrenaline (epinephrine) is the most important single drug in anaphylaxis. It reverses upper and lower airway oedema, causes bronchodilation, increases blood pressure, and causes peripheral vasoconstriction, reducing capillary leak. It should be given by the intramuscular route in most cases. The intravenous route should only be used by those experienced in this method, and with adrenaline at a concentration no greater than 1 in 10 000, with ECG monitoring. The prevalence of peanut allergy in childhood has tripled over the past decade and it now affects 1.5%. Up to 80% of children with this allergy react on the first apparent ingestion, suggesting previous occult sensitisation. The median age at onset is 2 years, and only 20% of young children with mild allergy can expect to grow out of it. A management plan for nut-allergic children which includes avoidance advice and a tailored patient-held self-treatment plan, together with regular follow-up, can reduce the number of further nut-induced reactions. An EpiPen should be carried by the child or held by the school. Future potential treatments include use of anti-IgE, and desensitisation with modified peanut allergen.

20.11 B: *Mycoplasma pneumoniae* pneumonia

Mycoplasma pneumoniae is a common cause of atypical pneumonia among school-age children. The clues in this history are malaise and headache, more common in *Mycoplasma* infection, together with the age of the child and lack of responsiveness to penicillin (*Mycoplasma* lacks a cell wall). *Pneumococcus* would also be a common pathogen in this context. Macrolide antibiotics are the treatment of choice. *Pneumocystis carinii* infection usually only affects children with a severe underlying immune deficiency, such as HIV, severe combined immunodeficiency syndrome (SCID) or DiGeorge syndrome, and after bone marrow transplantation.

20.12 E: pH study

This child presents with a picture of lower airway obstruction that is associated with feeds, suggesting the presence of gastro-oesophageal reflux disease, with or without aspiration. An H-type tracheo-oesophageal fistula could also cause this, although this is much rarer, and diagnosis requires a tube oesophogram (contrast injected under pressure). Flexible bronchoscopy is poor for excluding tracheo-oesophageal fistula, and ciliary brushing is used only for the diagnosis of primary ciliary dyskinesia. It would be sensible to screen for cystic fibrosis at a later stage.

20.13 D: Gastric aspirate cultures

The scenario describes a child with tuberculosis, the red lesions suggesting erythema nodosum. The presentation can be subtle, with few chest signs. The classic features of fever, lethargy and weight loss can be absent in children. Acid-fast bacilli are best obtained by gastric washings, usually on three successive mornings; bronchoalveolar lavage has a lower yield. The diagnosis can be confirmed by intradermal tuberculin testing. If there is a low likelihood of multi-resistant TB, initial treatment consists of isoniazid (for 6 months), rifampicin (6 months), and pyrazinamide (2 months). Monitor liver function tests and examine for peripheral neuropathy.

EMQ Answers

20.14 Management of pleural infection

1.   E: Ultrasound scan of the chest

New guidelines on the management of pleural infection in children were published by the British Thoracic Society (*Thorax* 2005; 60 [Suppl I]: i1–i21). If a pleural effusion is suspected, initial investigations include posteroanterior or anteroposterior X-rays. Obliteration of the costophrenic angle is the earliest sign of a pleural effusion, and a rim of fluid may be seen ascending the lateral chest wall (meniscus sign). A lateral chest radiograph rarely adds anything extra, and therefore should not be performed routinely. Chest ultrasonography can detect the presence of fluid in the pleural space, estimate the size of the effusion, differentiate free from loculated pleural fluid, determine the echogenicity of the fluid, and be used to guide the insertion of a chest drain or thoracocentesis, with the radiologist or radiographer marking the optimum site for drainage on the skin. Chest CT scans rarely add anything extra and, because of the additional radiation and costs, should not be performed routinely.

2.   F: Insertion of a small pigtail chest drain

Although many small parapneumonic effusions (thick fluid with loculations) will respond to antibiotics without the need for further intervention, effusions that are enlarging and/or compromising respiratory function in a febrile, unwell child need drainage. Repeated taps are not recommended. As there is no evidence that large-bore chest drains confer any advantage, small drains (including pigtail catheters) should be used whenever possible, to minimise patient discomfort and encourage mobilisation.

3.   D: Intrapleural fibrinolytics

Intrapleural fibrinolytic drugs have been shown to shorten the hospital stay, and are recommended for any complicated parapneumonic effusion (thick fluid with loculations) or empyema (overt pus). The recommended fibrinolytic is urokinase, which should be given twice daily for 3 days (6 doses in total) using 40 000 units in 40 mL 0.9% saline for children aged 1 year or more, and 10 000 units in 10 mL 0.9% saline for children younger than 1 year. Failure of chest-tube drainage, antibiotics and fibrinolytics should prompt early discussion with a thoracic surgeon. Potential surgical procedures include video-assisted thoracoscopic surgery and mini-thoracotomies, which only leave small scars. Decortication, which involves an open posterolateral thoracotomy and excision of the pleural rind with evacuation of pyogenic material, is a complicated procedure that leaves a large linear scar along the rib line, and is reserved for very severe cases.

20.15 Investigation of children with respiratory disease

1. G: Serum total and *Aspergillus*-specific IgE

Allergic bronchopulmonary aspergillosis is a recognised complication of cystic fibrosis and, less commonly, asthma. It arises as an overzealous allergic reaction to *Aspergillus* infection in the airways, leading to mucus impaction and airway narrowing. Patients present with dry cough, wheeze, and deterioration of lung function tests. It is suspected if total serum IgE is very high and *Aspergillus*-specific IgE and *Aspergillus* precipitins are increased. Wedge-shaped shadows are highly suggestive, although not always present. Treatment is with oral steroids and antifungal agents such as itraconazole, and may need to be medium- to long-term.

2. F: Rigid bronchoscopy

Foreign-body aspiration must always be considered in children who present with a monophonic wheeze and unilateral hyper-expansion on X-ray. Rigid, rather than flexible, bronchoscopy is required for removal of such objects.

3. C: Bronchoalveolar lavage

The girl is likely to have *Pneumocystis carinii* pneumonia. This extracellular parasite, recently named *Pneumocystis jirovecii* causes a relatively common opportunistic infection in patients with T-lymphocyte immunodeficiencies (eg HIV infection, CD40 ligand deficiency, or DiGeorge syndrome). Peak incidence is at age 3–6 months. Even when hypoxia is present, chest auscultation may reveal no crackles. Chest X-ray almost always shows bilateral diffuse alveolar shadowing. Bronchoalveolar lavage is the best method for isolating the organism, if it cannot be isolated from nasopharyngeal aspirate or sputum. Treatment is with high-dose co-trimoxazole (trimethoprim–sulfamethoxazole), pentamidine or dapsone. Children at risk of infection should receive prophylactic co-trimoxazole.

21. Rheumatology

Multiple True–False Questions

21.1   The following are complications of juvenile idiopathic arthritis:
- [ ] A   leg-length discrepancy
- [ ] B   benign joint hypermobility syndrome
- [ ] C   amyloidosis
- [ ] D   joint contractures
- [ ] E   blindness

21.2   Which of the following statements about auto-antibodies are true?
- [ ] A   anti-Ro antibody is associated with neonatal heart block
- [ ] B   anti-Ro antibody is associated with Sjögren syndrome
- [ ] C   anti-double-stranded DNA (dsDNA) antibody is highly specific for SLE
- [ ] D   anti-nuclear antibody (ANA) is usually positive in Kawasaki disease
- [ ] E   a positive rheumatoid factor is significant in reactive arthritis

21.3   Lyme disease:
- [ ] A   caused by the spirochaete, *Borrelia burgdorferi*
- [ ] B   has erythema marginatum as the characteristic rash
- [ ] C   must include a history of a tick bite to make the diagnosis
- [ ] D   associated with a facial nerve palsy
- [ ] E   arthritis is a common presenting feature

21.4   Arthritis is associated with the following conditions:
- [ ] A   fibromyalgia
- [ ] B   sarcoidosis
- [ ] C   sickle cell anaemia
- [ ] D   cystic fibrosis
- [ ] E   polyarteritis nodosa

21.5   The following are side-effects of methotrexate:
- [ ] A   nausea
- [ ] B   mouth ulcers
- [ ] C   transaminaemia
- [ ] D   skin rash
- [ ] E   leukopenia

21.6 Kawasaki disease is associated with which of the following?

☐ A   thrombocytopenia
☐ B   purulent conjunctivitis
☐ C   aseptic meningitis
☐ D   coronary artery aneurysms in 40%
☐ E   generalised lymphadenopathy

Best of Five Questions

21.7 A 2-year-old boy presents with a 7-week history of fever, with daily spikes of 40°C, and a pink rash that comes and goes with the temperature. He has had swelling of both wrists, both knees and both ankles for 7 weeks. He has generalised lymphadenopathy. Investigations reveal anaemia, with a high white cell count (WCC), increased platelets, and very high erythrocyte sedimentation rate and C-reactive protein (CRP). Anti-nuclear antibody (ANA), double-stranded DNA, and rheumatoid factor (RF) are negative. Which of the following is the MOST likely diagnosis?

☐ A   Systemic lupus erythematosus
☐ B   Acute lymphoblastic leukaemia
☐ C   Systemic-onset juvenile idiopathic arthritis
☐ D   Parvovirus infection
☐ E   Neuroblastoma

21.8 A 14-year-old boy with ulcerative colitis presents with a 6-month history of left hip pain. He has had early-morning stiffness of both knees and his left ankle for the past 3 months. On examination, he has decreased range of movement of his left hip, with swelling of both knees, both ankles and right elbow. He has tenderness of his sacroiliac joints. Investigations show: haemoglobin 11.5 g/dL (normal range [NR] 10.5–12.5 g/dL), WCC 18 × 10⁹/L (NR 5–15 × 10⁹/L), platelets 562 × 10⁹/L (NR 150–400 × 10⁹/L), erythrocyte sedimentation rate (ESR) 93 mm/h (NR < 15 mm/h), CRP 10 mg/dL (NR < 5 mg/dL); ANA negative; human leukocyte antigen (HLA) B27 positive. Which of the following is the MOST likely diagnosis?

☐ A   Polyarticular juvenile idiopathic arthritis
☐ B   Reactive arthritis
☐ C   Psoriatic arthritis
☐ D   Oligoarticular juvenile idiopathic arthritis
☐ E   Arthritis related to inflammatory bowel disease

21.9 A 12-year-old boy presents with pain in both heels for 3 months. He has also been to the GP with a painful red eye on several occasions. On examination, he has an effusion in his left knee, decreased range of movement in his right hip, and tenderness along the Achilles tendons and heel. His erythrocyte sedimentation rate is 100 mm/h (NR < 15 mm/h), C-reactive protein 45 mg/dL (NR < 5 mg/dL), full blood count normal, human leukocyte antigen (HLA) B27 positive. What is the MOST likely diagnosis?

☐ A Enthesitis-related juvenile idiopathic arthritis
☐ B Psoriatic arthritis
☐ C Oligoarticular juvenile idiopathic arthritis
☐ D Polyarticular juvenile idiopathic arthritis
☐ E Arthritis related to inflammatory bowel disease

21.10 A 4-year-old boy presents with a history of recurrent right knee pain for 4 weeks. He has developed a limp. Previously he was very active. He had two bouts of tonsillitis recently, neither of which required antibiotic treatment. There has been no fever or rash. Examination reveals a completely normal right knee, and the only abnormality is loss of internal rotation at the right hip, but no pain. What is the MOST likely diagnosis?

☐ A Oligoarticular juvenile idiopathic arthritis
☐ B Benign joint hypermobility syndrome
☐ C Enthesitis-related arthritis
☐ D Perthes' disease
☐ E Reactive arthritis

21.11 A 15-year-old girl has a 1-year history of a rash and a 6-month history of arthralgia. She was born in the UK. Both parents are from Jamaica. The raised erythematous rash had started on her right forearm and then spread to her chest, back and both legs. She did not have a rash on her face. The rash did not respond to long-term treatment with antifungal agents. She had developed shortness of breath in the past 3 weeks. There was no history of temperatures, and she did not have night sweats. No travel abroad. No weight loss. She had multiple erythematous, well-circumscribed skin lesions all over her body. Respiratory examination showed bilateral fine crepitations over the lower lung fields. She had swelling of both her ankles and knees, which had reduced range of movement. Ophthalmological examination showed uveitis. Investigations showed: normal ECG, negative Mantoux test, sputum culture negative for acid-fast bacilli with no subsequent growth, negative urine analysis, normal renal function; full blood count normal, ESR 28 mm/h (NR < 15 mm/h), CRP 25 mg/dL (NR < 5 mg/dL), creatine kinase (CK) and lactate dehydrogenase (LDH) normal, anti-nuclear antibody (ANA), rheumatoid factor (RF), extractable nuclear antigen (ENA) and autoimmune antibody screen all negative; normal complement levels, angiotensin-converting enzyme (ACE) 192 U/L (NR 20–90 U/L). What is the MOST likely diagnosis?

☐ A   Systemic lupus erythematosus
☐ B   Tuberculosis
☐ C   Sarcoidosis
☐ D   Wegener's granulomatosis
☐ E   Polyarticular juvenile idiopathic arthritis

21.12 A 9-year-old girl has a 2-month history of pain and swelling of her right foot, associated with a limp. There was no preceding illness or trauma. In the past month she had pain and swelling of her right thumb. Her mother has psoriasis. On examination, she has swelling of her right thumb, right big toe, right foot and right ankle. She has a plaque-like rash behind her left ear and on her umbilical region. What is the MOST likely diagnosis?

- [ ] A Oligoarticular juvenile idiopathic arthritis
- [ ] B Juvenile psoriatic arthritis
- [ ] C Juvenile dermatomyositis
- [ ] D Langerhans cell histiocytosis
- [ ] E Polyarticular juvenile idiopathic arthritis

21.13 A 14-year-old boy presented with a 3-month history of being unwell, with reduced appetite, excessive tiredness, and nausea at the sight of food. He developed a rash on his face and legs which lasted for 2–3 weeks then resolved. He had intermittent headaches and recently said he felt generally sore and that some of his joints were stiff in the mornings. On examination, he had some mouth ulcers, was thin and pale, had cervical and inguinal lymphadenopathy, no hepatosplenomegaly, bilateral knee swelling, and a faint red rash on his face. Cardiovascular and respiratory examination were normal. Laboratory results showed: haemoglobin 10.0 g/dL (NR 10.5–12.5 g/dL), white cell count 5.0×10^9/L (NR $5–15 \times 10^9$/L), lymphocytes 0.5×10^9/L (NR $1.5–7.0 \times 10^9$/L), platelets 128×10^9/L (NR $150–400 \times 10^9$/L), erythrocyte sedimentation rate 43 mm/h (NR < 15 mm/h), C-reactive protein < 3 mg/dL (NR < 5 mg/dL), anti-nuclear antibody 1 in 320 (positive), low C3 and C4 levels. What is the MOST likely diagnosis?

- [ ] A Juvenile dermatomyositis
- [ ] B Polyarteritis nodosa
- [ ] C Anorexia nervosa
- [ ] D Systemic lupus erythematosus
- [ ] E Hyperthyroidism

Extended Matching Questions

21.14 Theme: Rheumatology investigations

A   Blood film
B   Creatine kinase
C   Lactate dehydrogenase
D   C-reactive protein
E   Bone marrow aspirate
F   Anti-nuclear antibody (ANA)
G   Anti-double-stranded DNA antibody (dsDNA)
H   Coombs' test
I   Anti-phospholipid antibodies
J   Rheumatoid factor

For each of the following case scenarios, select the most useful investigation as the next step from those listed above. Each option may be used once, more than once, or not at all.

☐   1.   A 9-year-old girl presents with a 1-month history of fever, rash, tiredness, and painful joints. On examination, she has arthritis in both knees, but the rest of her joints are clinically normal. She has rash on her face. Investigations show: haemoglobin 7.5 g/dL (NR 10.5–12. g/dL), WCC 5.6 × 10^9/L (NR 5–15 × 10^9/L), lymphocytes 0.7 × 10^9/L (NR 1.5–7.0 × 10^9/L), platelets 135 × 10^9/L (NR 150–400 × 10^9/L), erythrocyte sedimentation rate 67 mm/h (NR < 15 mm/h); C-reactive protein 4 mg/dL (NR < 5 mg/dL), anti-nuclear antibody 1 in 2560 (strongly positive), low C3 levels, urine testing positive for proteinuria and haematuria, renal function normal, with normal blood pressure.

☐   2.   A 4-year-old girl presents with a 2-month history of bilateral elbow swelling and left knee swelling. She has had daily temperatures for the past week. She has been lethargic and has lost weight. On examination she is irritable, with generalised lymphadenopathy and hepatosplenomegaly. Investigations show: ESR 72 mm/h, CRP 123 mg/dL (NR < 5 mg/dL), anti-nuclear antibody negative. Full blood count shows: haemoglobin 8.2 g/dL (NR 10.5–12.5 g/dL), WCC 3.1 × 10^9/L (NR 5–15 × 10^9/L), platelets 88 × 10^9/L (NR 150–400 × 10^9/L).

☐   3.   A 6-year-old boy is seen in clinic with a 6-month history of painful swollen knees, with early-morning stiffness for 2 hours every day. There was no history of trauma. There was no history of preceding infection. He had no history of pain or stiffness in any other joints. He had a normal appetite and was growing well. He was otherwise well, and there was no significant family history. On examination, there was marked swelling of both knees, with fixed flexion of 5° on both sides, with quadriceps muscle wasting. The remainder of his joints and general examination were normal. Blood tests showed ESR 27 mm/h (NR < 15 mm/h) and normal full blood count.

21.15 Theme: Rheumatology diagnosis case studies

A   Systemic-onset juvenile idiopathic arthritis
B   Enthesitis-related arthritis
C   Oligoarticular juvenile idiopathic arthritis
D   Becker's muscular dystrophy
E   Psoriatic arthritis
F   Systemic lupus erythematosus
G   Juvenile dermatomyositis (JDM)
H   Meningococcal septicaemia
I   Henoch–Schönlein purpura
J   Viral myositis

For each of the following case scenarios, select the most likely diagnosis from those listed above. Each option may be used once, more than once, or not at all.

☐ 1. A 3-year-old boy presents with a 4-week history of tiredness and weakness. He is unable to lift his arms to help with being dressed or undressed. There were no other symptoms, apart from one episode of diarrhoea. No temperatures. In the past 10 days he has developed a rash around his eyes and on his chest. He had a peri-orbital rash, and a rash over his metacarpophalangeal joints of both hands. He had generalised muscle weakness and got up from the floor with a positive Gower manoeuvre. Full blood count and CRP were normal, ESR 23 mm/h, creatine kinase (CK) 5323 U/L (NR 30–200 U/L), and lactate dehydrogenase (LDH) 3183 U/L (NR 100–300 U/L).

☐ 2. A 14-year-old boy presents with an 8-week history of swelling of both knees, and a dry rash over his elbows and knees. His father has dry skin patches in his scalp. The boy also is found to have swelling of two of his toes. His GP has been treating him for a fungal infection of his nails.

☐ 3. A 5-year-old boy presents to A & E with a 24-hour history of a rash on both legs, including his buttocks. He had a sore throat a week ago, which is better now. On examination, he has the rash as described, and swollen ankles and knees. There is no other rash present. He is apyrexial, has normal observations and looks well. There was 1+ proteinuria on urine analysis.

MT–F Answers

21.1   Complications of juvenile idiopathic arthritis (JIA): A C D E

Because of the accelerated growth of an affected limb, especially if
untreated for a long period of time, a leg-length discrepancy can develop in
children with JIA. Joint contractures will develop if disease is untreated or
severe and aggressive. Amyloidosis can be a complication of all forms of
JIA, but is more common in systemic-onset juvenile idiopathic arthritis,
particularly after a long period of unremitting disease. Blindness is a
complication of untreated chronic anterior uveitis. Uveitis is particularly
associated with anti-nuclear antibody (ANA)-positive oligoarticular disease.
Ophthalmological screening for uveitis is performed in patients with JIA.
Benign joint hypermobility syndrome refers to patients with hypermobile
joints, and is not a complication of JIA.

21.2   Auto-antibodies: A B C

Certain antibodies are associated with certain autoimmune diseases:

- anti-Ro antibody   SLE, Sjögren syndrome, neonatal heart block
- anti-La antibody   Sjögren syndrome, occasionally SLE, rheumatoid
  arthritis
- anti-Sm antibody very specific for SLE, especially among West Indians
- anti-Scl-70   systemic sclerosis, scleroderma
- anti-Jo-1   dermatomyositis, juvenile dermatomyositis,
  interstitial lung disease

Anti-double-stranded DNA (dsDNA) is an aid to diagnosis; it is highly
specific for SLE, and an increase in the antibody titre usually precedes a
clinical flare of disease. ANA is not diagnostic or specific for any particular
disease. Rheumatoid factor is non-specific.

21.3   Lyme disease: A D

Lyme disease is caused by the spirochaete, *Borrelia burgdorferi*, transmitted
by the *Ixodes* tick. Erythema migrans is the distinctive rash. It starts as a red
macule at site of the tick bite and expands over days or weeks to form a
large well-circumscribed erythematous lesion with central sparing. Arthritis

is a rare and late complication. Clinical features of Lyme disease can be divided into early and late manifestations:

Early: days–weeks	Late: months–years
Erythema migrans	Acrodermatitis chronica atrophicans
Lymphocytoma	Radiculoneuritis
Lymphocytic meningitis	Encephalomyelitis
Facial palsy	Cardiomyopathy
Myopericarditis	Uveitis, keratitis
Conjunctivitis	Episodic arthritis
Flu-like illness	Chronic arthritis
Arthralgia	

21.4   Arthritis in childhood: B C D E

Fibromyalgia is an idiopathic chronic pain syndrome; there is no synovitis associated with this diagnosis. Arthritis can occur with all the other diseases. Causes of arthritis in childhood include:

Bacterial infections	Septic arthritis, tuberculosis, streptococcal
Viral infections	Rubella, mumps, adenovirus, coxsackie B, parvovirus
Other infections	*Mycoplasma*, *Borrelia burgdorferi* (Lyme disease), *Rickettsia*
Reactive arthritis	Streptococcal
Inflammatory bowel disease	Ulcerative colitis, Crohn's disease
Vasculitis	Henoch–Schönlein purpura, Kawasaki disease
Haematological	Haemophilia, sickle cell disease
Malignancy	Leukaemia, neuroblastoma
Inflammatory disorders	Juvenile idiopathic arthritis, juvenile dermatomyositis, SLE, scleroderma, mixed connective tissue disease
Other	Sarcoidosis

21.5   Side-effects of methotrexate: A B C E

Methotrexate is the disease-modifying drug used most frequently in paediatric rheumatology. It is used not only in juvenile idiopathic arthritis, but also in dermatomyositis and scleroderma, and in some patients with lupus. It can cause nausea that responds to antiemetics such as odansetron, or nausea can be avoided if it is administered by subcutaneous injection. It can cause mouth ulcers, and folic acid supplements are given to prevent this and other side-effects. Pulmonary fibrosis is said to occur in adults, but is not seen in paediatric practice. Liver enzymes can rise, but not usually resulting in liver fibrosis. Methotrexate can lower platelet or white cell counts, and occasionally haemoglobin. Rash is not usually a side-effect.

21.6   Kawasaki disease: C

Current diagnostic criteria for Kawasaki disease stipulate that the child must have a daily spiking high temperature for at least 5 days, with four of the following five features:

- bulbar conjunctival injection without exudates
- changes in oral mucosa: red cracked lips, red mouth and throat, strawberry tongue
- erythema and swelling of the hands and feet with subsequent peeling, usually after 3 weeks
- generalised erythematous rash, especially on the trunk
- cervical lymphadenopathy.

Five days of fever is necessary for the diagnosis. The conjunctiva is red, but not purulent. Thrombocytosis is seen, rather than thrombocytopenia. Aneurysms of the coronary artery and other large arteries are seen in 25% of patients. Cervical lymphadenopathy only (rather than generalised) is a diagnostic criterion.

Best of Five Answers

21.7   C: Systemic-onset juvenile idiopathic arthritis

These are all the classic findings in systemic-onset juvenile idiopathic arthritis. More than a 2-week history of spiking fevers is one of the criteria needed for the diagnosis. The rash is salmon-pink and can vary in intensity over the day, being prominent at times of fever. Generalised lymphadenopathy is a common feature. Arthritis has to be present for more than 6 weeks in systemic-onset juvenile idiopathic arthritis. Systemic lupus erythematosus usually has a positive anti-nuclear antibody and normal C-reactive protein. Platelets are usually normal or low in acute lymphoblastic leukaemia. The history is too prolonged for parvovirus, and rash is unusual in neuroblastoma, as is a high platelet count.

21.8   E: Arthritis related to inflammatory bowel disease

Arthritis can be the first presenting feature of inflammatory bowel disease such as Crohn's disease or ulcerative colitis, particularly in children with arthritis who are failing to thrive without any obvious cause. Erythema nodosum and mouth ulcers are associated features.

21.9   A: Enthesitis-related juvenile idiopathic arthritis

These are all classic findings for the diagnosis of enthesitis-related juvenile idiopathic arthritis. Onset is generally seen in a male child older than 6 years. Acute symptomatic uveitis can occur. HLA B27 is usually positive. Sacroiliac joint tenderness is typical. There may be a history of ankylosing spondylitis in a first-degree relative.

21.10 D: Perthes' disease

Perthes' disease is avascular necrosis of the femoral head. It is more common in boys of this age. Frequently, it presents with referred pain to the knee, rather than hip pain. The only sign on examination may be loss of internal rotation initially. There can be an associated synovitis. The history here is too short for oligoarticular juvenile idiopathic arthritis (6 weeks being necessary for the diagnosis), and the hip is almost never affected with this. The patient is probably hypermobile, given that he is good at gymnastics, but the range of movement would be increased, with often 90° of internal rotation, rather than the limited movement of this patient. The history is possible for reactive arthritis, but an irritable hip would not last for 4 weeks, and it is unusual in other reactive arthritides for the hip to be affected.

21.11 C: Sarcoidosis

Sarcoidosis in children has a typical triad of polyarthritis, rash and uveitis. Other clinical features include parotid swelling, weight loss, malaise, hepatosplenomegaly and lymphadenopathy. Serum angiotensin-converting enzyme (ACE) can be normal in up to 50% of patients. Diagnosis is made histopathologically with the presence of non-caseating granuloma on tissue biopsy. The arthritis is characterised by 'boggy' large-joint and tendon sheath effusions. Older children may have a presentation similar to that of the adult multi-system disease. The abnormal respiratory findings in this patient indicate lung parenchymal involvement. This can progress to irreversible fibrosis. The high ACE concentration adds to the diagnosis here. The lack of antibodies and normal FBC goes against SLE as a diagnosis. The negative Mantoux test and sputum culture help rule out TB.

21.12 B: Juvenile psoriatic arthritis

In psoriatic arthritis, the rash may or may not be coincident with arthritis. Nail pitting is seen in psoriasis. Typically, dactylitis, with swelling of one or more of the distal interphalangeal joints (fingers or toes) occurs in an asymmetric distribution. It can affect a few or many joints. Some patients can develop uveitis, so slit-lamp monitoring is needed. Some patients are positive for anti-nuclear antibody and have a family history of psoriasis. The condition responds well to methotrexate.

21.13 D: Systemic lupus erythematosus

This boy exhibits several features within the criteria of systemic lupus erythematosus: rash on his face likely to be malar rash, knee swelling indicating arthritis, mouth ulcers, lymphopenia, thrombocytopenia, and a positive anti-nuclear antibody (ANA). In 1997 the American College of Rheumatology published criteria for diagnosis, according to which a person shall be said to have systemic lupus erythematosus if any four or more of the following 11 criteria are present:

- malar rash
- discoid rash
- photosensitivity
- oral ulcers
- arthritis
- serositis (pleuritis **or** pericarditis)
- renal disorder (persistent proteinuria > 0.5 g/day **or** cellular casts)
- neurological disorder (seizures **or** psychosis)
- haematological disorder (haemolytic anaemia **or** leukopenia **or** lymphopenia **or** thrombocytopenia)
- immunological disorder (anti-phospholipid antibodies **or** anti-double-stranded DNA antibody to native double-stranded DNA **or** anti-Sm antibody to Smith nuclear antigen **or** false-positive serological test for syphilis)
- anti-nuclear antibody (abnormal titre).

EMQ Answers

21.14 Rheumatology investigations

1. G: Anti-double-stranded DNA antibody (dsDNA)

Double-stranded DNA antibodies are often found in high levels in systemic lupus erythematosus (SLE), and are especially likely to be found if there is renal disease. As they are specific to SLE, and within this list this is the most specific test to ask for to confirm the diagnosis.

2. E: Bone marrow aspirate

This child is pancytopenic. Acute leukaemia must be excluded and, although a blood film will usually be performed automatically, it is not a conclusive test, whereas a bone marrow aspirate is definitive.

3. F: Anti-nuclear antibody (ANA)

This child has two joints affected (oligoarticular juvenile idiopathic arthritis) and is otherwise systemically well. As the history is of 6 months' duration, this child needs an ophthalmological examination to exclude uveitis. Knowing his anti-nuclear antibody (ANA) status is therefore the most useful test. If he is ANA-positive, he is at high risk of uveitis and should be screened sooner.

21.15 Rheumatology diagnosis case studies

1. G: Juvenile dermatomyositis (JDM)

The features are all classic of juvenile dermatomyositis. The rash associated with juvenile dermatomyositis is a peri-orbital violacious colour, which can be associated with oedema, and spares the malar area. Gottron's papules occur on the extensor surfaces of fingers, and are red, raised papular lesions. They can also occur on the elbows, knees and ankle joints. If there is palatal weakness, it will lead to nasal speech. Creatine kinase levels can be normal or increased, but lactate dehydrogenase is often increased. Anti-nuclear antibody is only positive in a small percentage of patients. In Becker's muscular dystrophy, the creatine kinase is very high. There are not enough features for the diagnosis of lupus erythematosus. Viral myositis often affects the calf muscles, has an associated high creatine kinase, and would tend to have a more acute history.

2. E: Psoriatic arthritis

Psoriatic arthritis can present with few or several joints affected. It can occur without the classic psoriatic rash, but occasionally a psoriatic-like rash as described here can be seen. Dactylitis is a feature of psoriatic arthritis and is rarely seen in other types of juvenile arthritis. The father's dry scalp patches could possibly be psoriatic; a family history is often seen. The nail problem might be psoriatic and, typically, pitting is seen. In enthesitis-related arthritis, enthesitis and tendonitis are features – which are not seen in this patient. Enthesitis is inflammation at the site of tendon insertion into bones such as at the posterior heel.

3. I: Henoch–Schönlein purpura

Henoch–Schönlein purpura usually occurs after the age of 3 years, with a slight male predominance. It may be preceded by infection, particularly with haemolytic streptococci. The rash can evolve from urticarial lesions that develop into purpuric macules, typically on the legs, feet and buttocks. The arthritis, involving large joints, can be very painful but is usually transient. Abdominal pain is usually severe, and complications such as intussusception can occur. Immunoglobulin A complexes are seen in the skin and glomeruli if these are biopsied. Renal involvement is common, affecting up to 50% of cases in the acute phase, with up to 5% progressing to chronic renal failure. Non-steroidal anti-inflammatory drugs are used, and occasionally steroids in severe disease. As this child is well, with normal observations, he does not have meningococcal septicaemia.

22. Statistics

Multiple True–False Questions

22.1 Randomisation of patients to treatments within a trial ensures that

☐ A the patient is unaware of the treatment group to which they are assigned
☑ B each patient has an equal chance of being in any treatment group
☐ C the treatment group is known before consent is obtained
☐ D although individuals receive different treatments, each patient will be allocated to the treatment most likely to benefit them
☐ E differences between treatments will be significant

22.2 Observational studies

☑ A cannot be randomised
☐ B give more convincing evidence of true differences than experimental studies
☐ C are always large
☐ D can never be useful
☐ E must be blinded

22.3 The standard error of an estimate

☐ A is smaller for larger sample sizes
☐ B is a measure of the precision of that estimate
☐ C cannot be negative
☑ D depends on the average value of the sample
☑ E is used to construct confidence intervals

22.4 A *p* value

☑ A indicates the statistical significance of any differences seen in the sample(s)
☐ B lies between −1 and +1
☐ C is more useful than a confidence interval for interpreting results
☑ D is the probability of obtaining the current sample if the null hypothesis is true
☐ E indicates the clinical significance of any differences seen in the sample(s)

22.5 **Reflex times are measured in a group of children aged 5 to 15 years old. The correlation between reflex time and age is calculated as 0.76 (95% confidence interval 0.7 to 0.82). In this study**

- ☑ A the correlation coefficient is significantly different from zero
- ☐ B more measurements need to be made
- ☑ C there is a linear association between reflex times and age
- ☐ D the association is clinically important
- ☐ E older children tend to have slower reflex times

22.6 **Blood pressure is measured in two groups of people. Those receiving some treatment have blood pressures that are on average 6 mmHg lower than those in the untreated group. A *t*-test was applied and *p* = 0.02, 95% confidence interval for the difference (4.16 to 7.84) mmHg. It is true to say that**

- ☑ A the treatment should be introduced as it might be clinically relevant
- ☑ B the treatment must have improved blood pressure by at least 4.16 mmHg on average in the population
- ☐ C the difference observed would have occurred by chance 1 time in 20 if there really was no treatment effect
- ☐ D randomisation to groups was not successful
- ☐ E the *t*-test would not have been appropriate if the blood pressure measurements were skewed

22.7 **The power of a study**

- ☐ A varies between −1 and +1
- ☐ B can be calculated retrospectively
- ☐ C is the probability of correctly rejecting the null hypothesis when it is false
- ☑ D increases as the sample size is increased
- ☐ E is larger the greater the difference that is to be detected

Best of Five Questions

22.8 In children with renal failure, a study shows that vitamin D
levels are found to be severely depleted ($p < 0.0001$). Which is
the MOST appropriate course of action based on this study?

- ☐ A Introduce vitamin D supplementation as standard practice
- ☑ B Consider extent of depletion, clinical implications, costs of
  supplementation and make a decision based on these
- ☐ C Re-analyse the data, taking into account the ages of the children
- ☐ D Carry out a further study of greater size
- ☐ E Do nothing

22.9 Cirrhotic children aged 6–10 years old are randomised to a new
dietary regimen or standard advice. After 2 years their height
standard deviation (SD) scores are compared. The group allocated
to the new diet have a higher mean SD score for height
(difference 0.2, 95% confidence interval [–0.8 to 1.2]) but this
difference is non-significant ($p = 0.52$). An improvement of
0.2 SD scores over a 2-year period would be considered clinically
important in this group of children. Which is the MOST
appropriate course of action based on this study?

- ☐ A Do nothing further – the study has shown the new diet is not
  statistically significantly better than current practice
- ☑ B Re-analyse the data using non parametric methods
- ☐ C Follow the children for longer to try and obtain statistical as well as
  clinical significance
- ☐ D Carry out a trial of a larger size to obtain a more precise estimate of
  the effect of the new diet compared with standard advice
- ☐ E Introduce the new diet as standard practice – the average
  improvement is clinically important

22.10 Haemoglobin measurements were made in small groups of
children with five different syndromes. In order to assess
whether there are differences between the groups that are
unlikely to have occurred by chance, which one of the following
is MOST appropriate?

- ☑ A A further study of much larger size
- ☐ B Analysis of variance comparing means between the groups
- ☐ C The data should be plotted according to syndromic group
- ☐ D Mann–Whitney U-tests between each pair of syndromic groups
- ☐ E Non-parametric analysis of variance comparing medians between
  groups (Kruskal–Wallis)

22.11 What is the BEST reason why concurrent control groups are useful when performing studies?

☑ A They allow the use of statistical tests for the comparison of two groups (eg two-sample t-tests)

☐ B They help to ensure that any differences seen are due to the treatment or disease being studied

☐ C They allow the study to be blinded

☐ D They help boost the overall numbers studied

☐ E They are better than historical controls

22.12 Which of the following applies MOST to a reference range for CD4 counts in childhood?

☑ A The study should be based on large numbers of children

☐ B The study needs to be age-related

☐ C It is useful for assessing children with known disease

☐ D It allows the CD4 counts of individual children to be compared with what is expected for normal children of that age

☐ E It does not give the sensitivity of low CD4 count in detecting disease

22.13 Intelligence (IQ) assessments and heights are measured in a group of healthy 7-year-olds. To investigate whether there is a meaningful, statistically significant relationship, which of the following is MOST appropriate?

☑ A The correlation coefficient should be calculated

☐ B A regression analysis should be used and the regression coefficient presented with confidence interval

☐ C A p value must be obtained

☐ D More assessments could be made

☐ E Heights should be expressed as SD (standard deviation) scores

Extended Matching Questions

22.14 Theme: Significance tests

A   Two-sample t-test
B   Paired t-test
C   Mann–Whitney U-test
D   One-way analysis of variance
E   Kruskal–Wallis analysis of variance
F   Regression analysis
G   Correlation coefficient
H   Chi-square

For each of the following study scenarios, choose the most appropriate statistical test from the list above to analyse the data. Each option may be used once, more than once, or not at all.

1. Blood pressure measurements are made in a group of children with pituitary hormone disorders and in age- and sex-matched control pairs. The study aims to investigate whether pituitary hormone disorders are associated with altered blood pressure.

2. Developmental tests are applied to determine whether children who were admitted to intensive care in the neonatal period are more likely to have delayed development at age 5 years than those who were not.

3. Blood pressures (assumed normally distributed) are compared between 5-year-olds from four different, clearly defined racial backgrounds.

22.15 Theme: Interpreting trial results

A   The difference is statistically and clinically significant; the new cream should not be introduced
B   The difference is statistically significant but the difference is clinically small; the new cream should be introduced
C   A larger study is required to determine whether it is worth introducing the new cream
D   The difference between the creams is both statistically and clinically significant; the new cream should be introduced
E   The difference is statistically significant but the difference is not of clinical importance and the new cream should not be introduced
F   The study provides enough evidence to discount the usefulness of the new cream
H   The study is invalidated by the drop-outs
I   The results cannot be interpreted because the analysis used was inappropriate

A randomised controlled trial is used to compare the effectiveness of a new cream (T) for treating eczema compared with the current alternative cream (C) for children aged 5–10 years of age. Severity is rated on a 0 (no rash) to 10 (severe rash) scale. An average fall of 2 points on the severity scale attributable to the new cream would be deemed of clinical importance and worth changing to the new cream to achieve. For the following study results choose the most appropriate interpretation from the list above. Each option may be used once, more than once, or not at all.

1. Those allocated to the new cream have an average rating of 5.4 compared with 7.8 for those on the current alternative (95% confidence interval for the difference [−3.6 to −1.2], $p < 0.0005$).
2. Those allocated to the new cream have an average rating of 5.4 compared with 7.8 for those on the current alternative (95% confidence interval for the difference [−6.0 to 1.2], $p = 0.23$).
3. Of the 40 children allocated to the two creams, 30 who used the new cream had an average severity rating of 5.4. The 50 children who used the current treatment (40 randomised to this treatment plus the 10 who did not use the new cream but reverted to the current cream) had an average rating of 7.8. The 95% confidence interval for the mean fall in severity rating (−2.4) was (−3.6 to −1.2), $p < 0.0005$.

MT–F Answers

22.1 Randomisation to treatments in a trial: B

Participants should be randomised to groups to remove any potential bias, meaning that each patient has the same chance of being assigned to either of the groups, regardless of their personal characteristics. Randomisation aims to ensure that the treatment groups are similar, apart from the treatment under study, so that any differences in outcome are more easily attributable to being causally related to treatment. It is the procedure of blinding – not randomisation – that ensures that individuals do not know which groups they are in. Randomisation should take place after consent is obtained. Randomisation does not ensure that differences in treatments will be significant.

22.2 Observational studies: A

In observational studies the groups being compared are already defined and the study merely observes what happens. Because groups (different diseases or different treatments) are already determined and known they cannot be blind or randomised. The size of the sample that is studied is determined by the researcher and may be small. If a difference is found in an observational study then it is more likely to be due to confounding factors than it is in an experimental trial, because the groups were determined before the study. A difference found with an experimental design is more likely to result from the treatment than it is in an observational study. Despite the potential for confounding, observational studies can provide useful information. Interpretation of the results should take into account the limitations of the design.

22.3 Standard error of an estimate: A B C E

The standard error is a measure of how precisely the sample value approximates the true population value. For continuous data it is calculated as the standard deviation divided by the square root of the sample size. Confidence intervals can be constructed around the sample estimate using the standard error. Precision will obviously be greater or better for larger sample sizes and we can also see this from the formula for calculating standard error. (The standard deviation is divided by the square root of the sample size, so as the sample size increases we divide by a larger number, and the standard error will be smaller, indicating greater or better precision.) Also, since the standard deviation is always positive, the standard error must also be positive. Although it depends on the spread of the values around the average (ie the standard deviation) it does not depend on the average itself, being a measure of the precision of that average.

22.4   p value: A D

The p value is the probability of obtaining the current sample if the null hypothesis were true. It gives a measure of the statistical significance of any differences seen. As it is a probability it can range from 0 (no probability/never happens) to 1 (certainty/always happens) but cannot be negative. The p value gives an indication of how likely one particular hypothesised value is to be true, whereas the confidence interval gives the range of hypothesised values with which the sample is compatible. Hence confidence intervals give much more information and enable clinical interpretation of the results. The p value gives statistical significance, but clinical significance will depend on other factors such as inconvenience associated with treatment, level of improvement, or difference and costs.

22.5   Reflex times: A C

The correlation coefficient gives a measure of linear association between reflex times and age. Zero indicates no linear association; the closer the value is to +1 or –1, the stronger the linear association. For this sample, the value is 0.76, which indicates some linear association. The coefficient is positive and this shows that age and reflex time both increase together (that is, older children have longer reflex times). The confidence interval for the correlation (0.7 to 0.82) does not contain zero and the correlation is therefore significantly different from zero. Whether or not more measurements need to be made depends on whether the precision obtained for the estimate is suitable for whatever purpose it was made. The association is statistically significant; whether it is clinically important depends on additional factors.

22.6   Treatment for blood pressure: E

The difference observed is statistically significant and would have occurred by chance 2 times in 100 (since $p = 0.02$) or 1 time in 50 if there really were no treatment effect. We cannot tell from the information given whether or not randomisation was successful. The sample is compatible with an average fall in blood pressure of between 4.16 and 7.84 mmHg. We are 95% confident that the population average fall lies within this interval, but it may not (in fact, 5% of the time it will not). Statistical significance does not necessarily imply clinical significance or relevance. The *t*-test is not valid if the measurements are not normally distributed. Skewed data are not normally distributed.

22.7   Power of a study: B C D E

The power of a study is the probability (usually expressed as a percentage) of correctly rejecting the null hypothesis when it is false. As it is a probability it must lie between 0 and 1 (or 0 and 100% when expressed as a percentage). The greater the difference to be detected, the greater the chance that the study will find it; hence the power is larger for bigger differences. The larger the sample size, the greater the power to detect a difference of a given size. Power is usually calculated at the commencement of a study. Sample size is often based on achieving a given power to detect differences of clinically important magnitude. Sample size estimation is based on unknown quantities and the estimations of power can be made once those quantities have been determined from the sample data. Hence power can be calculated retrospectively.

Best of Five Answers

22.8   B: Consider extent of depletion, clinical implications, costs of supplementation and make a decision based on these

There is a statistically significant difference as shown by the *p* value. We are not told who the renal failure children were compared with to get that value. Was this concurrent healthy controls or an established reference range? How we interpret the results will depend on who the comparison was made with. The difference seen is statistically significant but this may or may not be associated with a clinically important difference – although the fact that the question states that values are 'severely' depleted suggests a clinically relevant reduction has occurred. There may or may not be other factors, such as age, that need to be taken into account when interpreting the results. The study was presumably undertaken to answer some research question, the answer to which would inform clinical practice. Therefore we do not expect to do nothing after obtaining the trial results. On the other hand, we do not want to introduce (or even trial) supplementation without first considering the clinical relevance and implications for the reduction found. The *p* value shows that the study is large enough that the observed difference cannot be attributed to chance. Hence, the most correct answer is B.

22.9 D: Carry out a trial of a larger size to obtain a more precise estimate of the effect of the new diet compared with standard advice

The average improvement seen is clinically relevant so we would not just want to discount the information because it is statistically non-significant. The confidence interval for the difference is wide and shows that the data are compatible with the new dietary regimen, having no effect or an adverse effect on height, and also with clinically relevant improvements (up to 1.2 SD scores). Because the diet could be associated with a detrimental or zero effect based on the study results, it would not be reasonable to introduce it as standard purely because the average effect is good. The children could be followed for longer to see whether the effect becomes larger and statistically significant but this would not answer the question of whether an improvement can be seen over 2 years. SD scores are usually normally distributed, so it is unlikely – although not impossible – that non-parametric methods would be needed. The normality of the scores should have been verified prior to parametric testing. A larger trial would enable a more precise estimate of the effect of the new diet over a 2-year period to be obtained and this would be the best course of action (so D is the most correct answer).

22.10 E: Non-parametric analysis of variance comparing medians between groups (Kruskal–Wallis)

The groups are small, so it is likely that parametric methods are not appropriate. Before embarking on a formal analysis of the differences, the haemoglobin measurements should be plotted according to syndrome group. This plot will allow some assessment of the normality of the measurements. Testing between pairs of groups will enable significant differences to be identified but it does rely on multiple tests and the p values obtained will not be valid without adjustment. It would be preferable to perform one overall test of the significance of the differences observed between groups. It may be that the study is not large enough to identify differences of clinical importance and a larger sample is required. This will become apparent from the plot, significance test and confidence intervals.

22.11 B: They help to ensure that any differences seen are due to the treatment or disease being studied

If there is no control group then it will not be possible to say whether any effects/outcomes seen in the diseased or treated group are due to the disease or treatment, so a control group is necessary. If a historical control group (a group previously measured/assessed) is used then we cannot be sure that any difference is not due to factors that have changed over time (for example, improvement in diet or clinical care). Concurrent controls are therefore preferable. Using concurrent controls will remove some of the potential confounders. We want the controls to be similar to the treatment/disease group so that any differences observed are more likely to be causally attributed to the treatment or disease. If the groups are blind to treatment then treatment knowledge does not differ between groups and so this is a similarity that we want to have (where ethically and feasibly possible).

22.12 D: It allows the CD4 counts of individual children to be compared with what is expected for normal children of that age

A reference range aims to give information on the values of CD4 found among normal, non-diseased children. It consists of a series of centile values. Since CD4 count changes throughout childhood, the range should be age-related. In order to construct precise ranges, quite large groups of children will be needed as we are often interested in extreme centiles (the 5th and beyond). Often the 5th centile is used as a cut-off to define abnormality or cause for further investigation. By definition, 5% of normal healthy individuals will lie on or below the 5th centile. Hence the specificity of a test which uses the 5th centile as a cut-off will be 95% and 95% of those without disease (healthy, normal children like those on whom the reference was based) will have values above the 5th centile and will test 'negative'. The sensitivity of a reference range to detect disease will vary according to the disease. The purpose of the reference range is to allow the CD4 counts of individual children to be compared with what is expected for normal children of that age. If the aim was to compare a group of children with disease with a group of non-diseased children, then these non-diseased children should be concurrently measured. Reference ranges are not recommended as a substitute for control groups in trials, rather as assessment tools for individual children. The most correct answer is therefore D.

22.13 B: A regression analysis should be used and the regression coefficient presented with confidence interval

Firstly the data should be plotted in a scatterplot of IQ against height. The correlation coefficient could be calculated to estimate significance of any observed association. The relationship could be further quantified by regressing IQ scores on height. This will give a measure of the extent to which IQ changes with height and is much more informative than the correlation coefficient alone. The extent to which the two are related is given by the regression coefficient. Presenting the regression coefficient with a confidence interval shows the range of population scenarios the current sample is compatible with. If the confidence interval is wide then we may decide that a larger sample needs to be taken to obtain a more precise estimate of the relationship. The statistical significance of the observed difference is given by the p value. Since the sample are all 7 years old it is unlikely that expressing their heights as SD scores will make any difference to the results. If the children were over a wider age range and we wanted to remove age as a potential confounder in the comparison of IQ and height, then expressing heights as SD scores would do this.

EMQ Answers

22.14 Significance tests

1. B: Paired t-test

There are two groups of children (those with pituitary hormone disorders and their age–sex-matched control pairs). Hence a two-sample test for comparison between groups is appropriate (two-sample t-test, paired t-test, Mann–Whitney U-test, or chi-square). Outcomes are continuous numeric (blood pressure) and it is the within-pair difference that will be analysed (blood pressure for child with disorder, minus blood pressure for age- and sex-matched pair). Hence the test must be appropriate for continuous outcome data (that is, not chi-square). Since it is within-pair differences that are to be analysed (so two-sample t-test and Mann–Whitney U-test inappropriate), these are likely to be normally distributed. The appropriate test to use is the paired t-test.

2. H: Chi-square

There are two groups of children (those admitted to intensive care and those who were not). Hence a two-sample test for comparison between groups is appropriate (two-sample t-test, paired t-test, Mann–Whitney U-test or chi-square). Outcome is binary, that is categoric, with two categories (developmentally delayed: yes/no). The proportion with developmental delay is to be compared between those admitted to intensive care or not. The appropriate test for comparing proportions between two groups is chi-square.

3. D: One-way analysis of variance

There are four groups of children to be compared (from different racial backgrounds). Hence a test for simultaneous comparison between more than two groups is appropriate (one-way analysis of variance, Kruskal–Wallis analysis of variance or chi-square). The outcome (blood pressure) is continuous (hence chi-square is not appropriate) and normally distributed and so parametric testing should be used (eg one-way analysis of variance).

22.15 Interpreting trial results

For all sections, A cannot be correct. If the new cream is found to be both statistically and clinically significant then this means that the difference observed is unlikely to be due to chance and is also large enough to make it clinically relevant. The study shows the average difference attributable to the new cream must be large enough to be of clinical importance after taking into account all other factors (cost, ease of use, problems associated with introducing new treatment). Hence if the new cream is statistically and clinically significant then it should be introduced and so stem A can never be true.

1. C: A larger study is required to determine whether it is worth introducing the new cream

The difference is statistically significant because the p value (< 0.0005) is small. The average fall of 2.4 points on the severity scale is larger than deemed sufficient to be of clinical importance. However, the confidence interval shows that the data are compatible with a difference of between 1.2 and 3.6 points. An average fall of 1.2 would not be deemed clinically important enough to warrant changing to the new cream. So the data are compatible with outcomes that are synonymous with differing courses of action. For a fall of 1.2 to less than 2 points on average, the cream would not be introduced, whereas an average fall of between 2 and 3.6 would lead to introduction of the cream. A larger study needs to be done to reduce the width of the confidence interval and gain a more precise estimate of the value of the new cream.

2. C: A larger study is required to determine whether it is worth introducing the new cream

The difference is statistically non-significant because the p value (0.23) is not small. The confidence interval shows that the sample data are compatible with an average change of anywhere between a 6-point drop in favour of the new cream and it making the rash 1.2 points worse on average. Hence we cannot discount scenarios that would lead to introduction of the new cream (ie a fall of between 6 and 2 on average on the severity scale). Neither can we discount the fact that the new cream does not have a clinically important effect (difference may be less than 2 points and the p value and confidence interval both show data are compatible with no difference between the creams). Hence a larger study needs to be done to distinguish between differences of clinical relevance and not.

3. **I: The results cannot be interpreted because the analysis used was inappropriate**

The difference, confidence intervals and p value are the same as in (1). The observed difference is statistically significant but may or may not be of a clinically relevant magnitude. However, the children allocated to the new cream, but not using it, have been combined with those in the other allocation group. Hence the groups are no longer randomly selected. Those who changed treatment from their allocation may differ in some way that biases the results. The data should have been analysed on an intention-to-treat basis (that is, outcomes compared according to allocated group, rather than according to the treatment actually used). This flaw in the analysis makes it impossible to interpret the results as we cannot assess the extent of any bias.

Index